T0131142

The Physiotherapist's Pocketbook

Content Strategist: Poppy Garraway
Content Development Specialist: Veronika Watkins
Senior Project Manager: Kamatchi Madhavan
Designer: Brian Salisbury

The Physiotherapist's Pocketbook

Essential facts at your fingertips

THIRD EDITION

Karen Kenyon MRes, BSc (Hons), BA (Hons), MCSP
Sussex Partnership NHS Foundation Trust, UK

Jonathan Kenyon MSc, PGCert (NMP), BSc (Hons), MMACP, MCSP
Sussex Partnership NHS Foundation Trust, UK

ELSEVIER

Edinburgh London New York Oxford Philadelphia St Louis Sydney Toronto 2018

ELSEVIER

© 2018 Elsevier Limited. All rights reserved.

First edition 2004
Second edition 2009

ISBN 978-0-7020-5506-5
e-book 978-07020-7798-2

British Library Cataloguing in Publication Data
A catalogue record for this book is available from the British Library

Library of Congress Cataloging in Publication Data
A catalog record for this book is available from the Library of Congress

Notices

Practitioners and researchers must always rely on their own experience and knowledge in evaluating and using any information, methods, compounds or experiments described herein. Because of rapid advances in the medical sciences, in particular, independent verification of diagnoses and drug dosages should be made. To the fullest extent of the law, no responsibility is assumed by Elsevier, authors, editors or contributors for any injury and/or damage to persons or property as a matter of products liability, negligence or otherwise, or from any use or operation of any methods, products, instructions, or ideas contained in the material herein.

The Publisher

your source for books,
journals and multimedia
in the health sciences

www.elsevierhealth.com

  Working together
to grow libraries in
developing countries

The
publisher's
policy is to use
paper manufactured
from sustainable forests

www.elsevier.com • www.bookaid.org

Printed in China

Last digit is the print number: 9   8   7

CONTENTS

Eighteen years ago we were newly qualified physiotherapists working in busy London teaching hospitals when we came up with an idea that would later become *The Physiotherapist's Pocketbook*. Like hundreds of physiotherapists before us, we prepared for clinical placements and rotations by compiling pocket-sized reference notes that we could access quickly and easily when we needed to check something. As we made our way through our rotations these "crib sheets" slowly grew into a compendium of key information covering all the core areas of physiotherapy, forming the basis of the *Pocketbook*.

When we first wrote the *Pocketbook* we never thought we would be writing the third edition 14 years later. We have been overwhelmed by the favourable response to the previous two editions and have endeavoured to ensure this new edition provides a relevant and up-to-date resource that is as comprehensive and useful as possible to all clinicians. It is beyond the scope and size of the book to cover the more specialist areas of physiotherapy, but we hope that its sections on anatomy, neuromusculoskeletal examination, neurology, respiratory, pharmacology and pathology and the supporting appendices are broad enough to fulfil its main purpose – to provide quick and easy access to essential clinical information during everyday clinical practice.

A project of this size would not be possible without the support of our publishing team at Elsevier who have guided us throughout the writing and production process. In addition, we have been fortunate to work alongside a large number of colleagues, students and academics who have provided invaluable encouragement and advice. If we could name them all this would definitely not be a pocket-sized book, but we would like to say a special thanks to all our colleagues and friends at East Sussex Healthcare NHS Trust, Brighton and Sussex Hospital NHS Trust and The Sussex Musculoskeletal Partnership (Central and East).

This book is dedicated to our wonderful children, Jack and Eva, who have had to put up with more "physio stuff" than any child should ever be subjected to.

Neuromusculoskeletal anatomy

Musculoskeletal anatomy illustrations

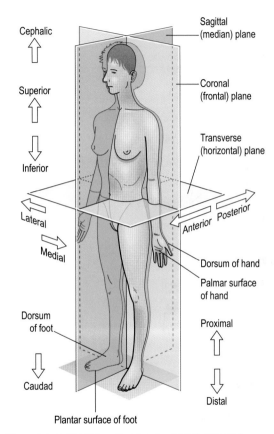

Figure 1.1 Anatomical position showing cardinal planes and directional terminology.

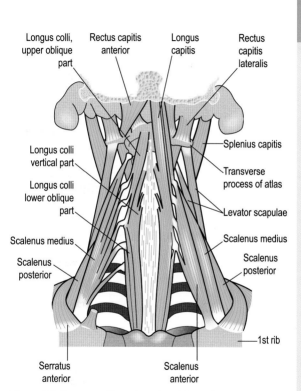

Longus colli, upper oblique part

Rectus capitis anterior

Longus capitis

Rectus capitis lateralis

Longus colli vertical part

Longus colli lower oblique part

Scalenus medius

Scalenus posterior

Splenius capitis

Transverse process of atlas

Levator scapulae

Scalenus medius

Scalenus posterior

Serratus anterior

Scalenus anterior

1st rib

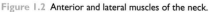

Figure 1.2 Anterior and lateral muscles of the neck.

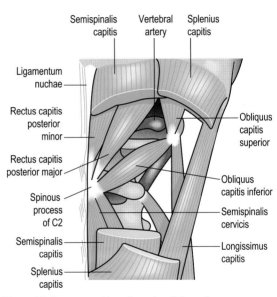

Figure 1.3 Posterior and lateral muscles of the neck.

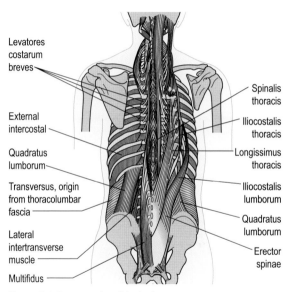

Levatores costarum breves

External intercostal

Quadratus lumborum

Transversus, origin from thoracolumbar fascia

Lateral intertransverse muscle

Multifidus

Spinalis thoracis

Iliocostalis thoracis

Longissimus thoracis

Iliocostalis lumborum

Quadratus lumborum

Erector spinae

Figure 1.4 Deep muscles of the back.

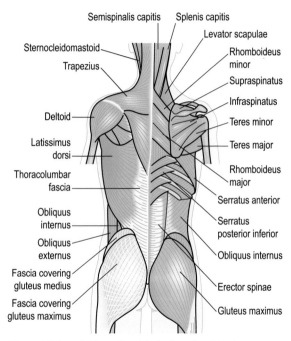

Semispinalis capitis

Splenis capitis

Levator scapulae

Sternocleidomastoid

Rhomboideus minor

Trapezius

Supraspinatus

Infraspinatus

Deltoid

Teres minor

Latissimus dorsi

Teres major

Thoracolumbar fascia

Rhomboideus major

Serratus anterior

Obliquus internus

Serratus posterior inferior

Obliquus externus

Obliquus internus

Fascia covering gluteus medius

Erector spinae

Fascia covering gluteus maximus

Gluteus maximus

Figure 1.5 Superficial muscles of the back, neck and trunk.

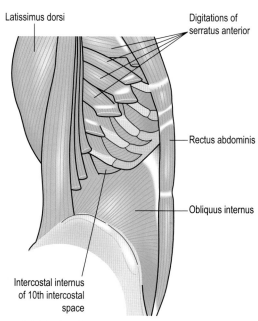

Latissimus dorsi

Digitations of
serratus anterior

Rectus abdominis

Obliquus internus

Intercostal internus
of 10th intercostal
space

Figure 1.6 Muscles of the right side of the trunk.

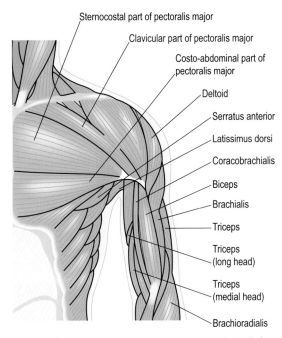

Sternocostal part of pectoralis major

Clavicular part of pectoralis major

Costo-abdominal part of pectoralis major

Deltoid

Serratus anterior

Latissimus dorsi

Coracobrachialis

Biceps

Brachialis

Triceps

Triceps (long head)

Triceps (medial head)

Brachioradialis

Figure 1.7 Superficial muscles of the anterior chest and arm. Left side.

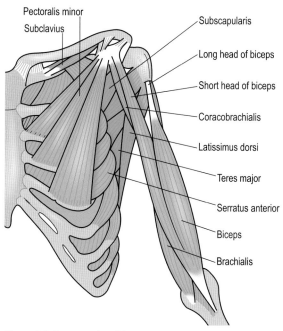

Figure 1.8 Deep muscles of the anterior chest and upper arm. Left side.

Pectoralis minor

Subclavius

Subscapularis

Long head of biceps

Short head of biceps

Coracobrachialis

Latissimus dorsi

Teres major

Serratus anterior

Biceps

Brachialis

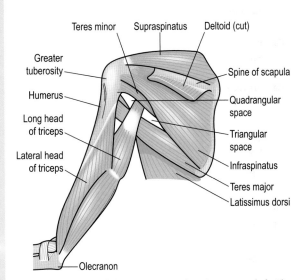

Figure 1.9 Muscles of the posterior scapula and upper arm. Left side.

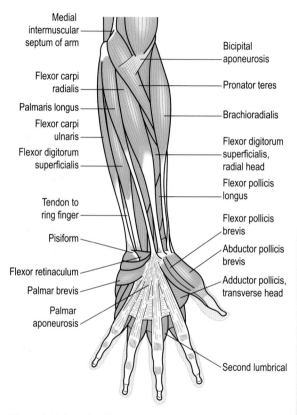

Medial intermuscular septum of arm

Flexor carpi radialis

Palmaris longus

Flexor carpi ulnaris

Flexor digitorum superficialis

Tendon to ring finger

Pisiform

Flexor retinaculum

Palmar brevis

Palmar aponeurosis

Bicipital aponeurosis

Pronator teres

Brachioradialis

Flexor digitorum superficialis, radial head

Flexor pollicis longus

Flexor pollicis brevis

Abductor pollicis brevis

Adductor pollicis, transverse head

Second lumbrical

Figure 1.10 Superficial flexors of the left forearm.

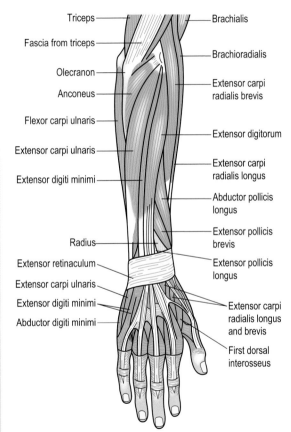

Triceps

Fascia from triceps

Olecranon

Anconeus

Flexor carpi ulnaris

Extensor carpi ulnaris

Extensor digiti minimi

Radius

Extensor retinaculum

Extensor carpi ulnaris

Extensor digiti minimi

Abductor digiti minimi

Brachialis

Brachioradialis

Extensor carpi radialis brevis

Extensor digitorum

Extensor carpi radialis longus

Abductor pollicis longus

Extensor pollicis brevis

Extensor pollicis longus

Extensor carpi radialis longus and brevis

First dorsal interosseus

Figure 1.11 Superficial extensors of the right forearm.

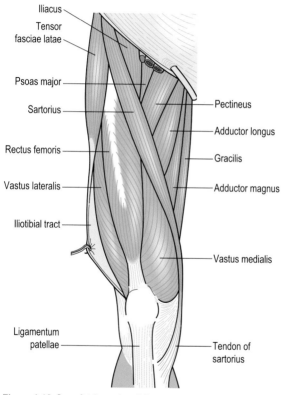

Iliacus

Tensor fasciae latae

Psoas major

Sartorius

Rectus femoris

Vastus lateralis

Iliotibial tract

Ligamentum patellae

Pectineus

Adductor longus

Gracilis

Adductor magnus

Vastus medialis

Tendon of sartorius

Figure 1.12 Superficial muscles of the anterior right thigh.

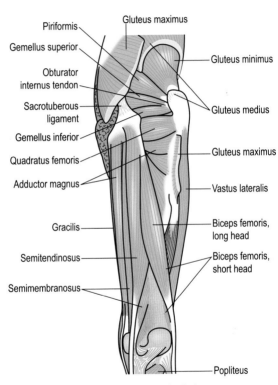

Piriformis

Gemellus superior

Obturator
internus tendon

Sacrotuberous
ligament

Gemellus inferior

Quadratus femoris

Adductor magnus

Gracilis

Semitendinosus

Semimembranosus

Gluteus maximus

Gluteus minimus

Gluteus medius

Gluteus maximus

Vastus lateralis

Biceps femoris,
long head

Biceps femoris,
short head

Popliteus

Figure 1.13 Muscles of the posterior right thigh.

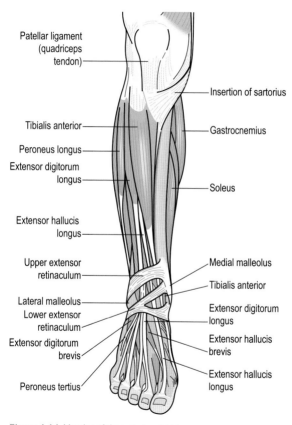

Patellar ligament (quadriceps tendon)

Insertion of sartorius

Tibialis anterior

Gastrocnemius

Peroneus longus

Extensor digitorum longus

Soleus

Extensor hallucis longus

Upper extensor retinaculum

Medial malleolus

Tibialis anterior

Lateral malleolus

Lower extensor retinaculum

Extensor digitorum longus

Extensor hallucis brevis

Extensor digitorum brevis

Peroneus tertius

Extensor hallucis longus

Figure 1.14 Muscles of the anterior right leg.

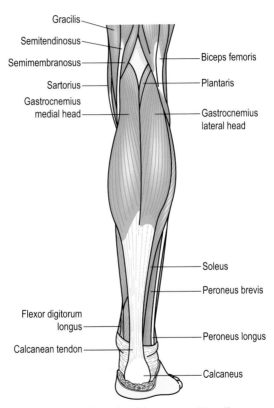

Gracilis

Semitendinosus

Semimembranosus

Sartorius

Gastrocnemius
medial head

Biceps femoris

Plantaris

Gastrocnemius
lateral head

Soleus

Peroneus brevis

Flexor digitorum
longus

Peroneus longus

Calcanean tendon

Calcaneus

Figure 1.15 Superficial muscles of the posterior right calf.

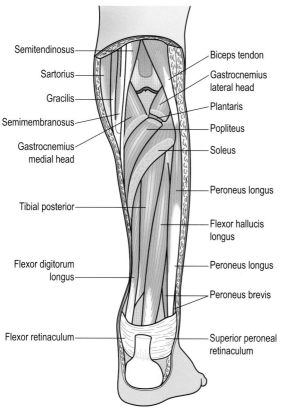

Semitendinosus

Sartorius

Gracilis

Semimembranosus

Gastrocnemius
medial head

Tibial posterior

Flexor digitorum
longus

Flexor retinaculum

Biceps tendon

Gastrocnemius
lateral head

Plantaris

Popliteus

Soleus

Peroneus longus

Flexor hallucis
longus

Peroneus longus

Peroneus brevis

Superior peroneal
retinaculum

Figure 1.16 Deep muscles of the posterior right calf.

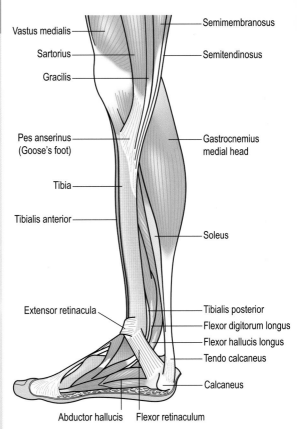

Vastus medialis

Sartorius

Gracilis

Pes anserinus
(Goose's foot)

Tibia

Tibialis anterior

Extensor retinacula

Abductor hallucis

Semimembranosus

Semitendinosus

Gastrocnemius
medial head

Soleus

Tibialis posterior

Flexor digitorum longus

Flexor hallucis longus

Tendo calcaneus

Calcaneus

Flexor retinaculum

Figure 1.17 Muscles of the medial right leg.

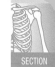

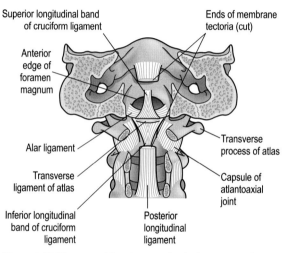

Superior longitudinal band of cruciform ligament

Ends of membrane tectoria (cut)

Anterior edge of foramen magnum

Alar ligament

Transverse process of atlas

Transverse ligament of atlas

Capsule of atlantoaxial joint

Inferior longitudinal band of cruciform ligament

Posterior longitudinal ligament

Figure 1.18 Ligaments of the atlanto-axial and atlanto-occipital joints.

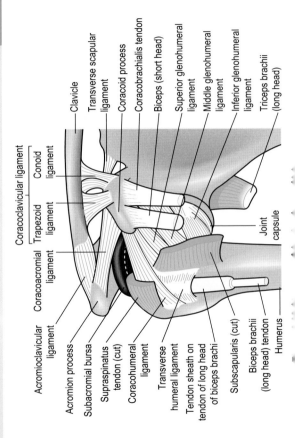

- Clavicle
- Transverse scapular ligament
- Coracoid process
- Coracobrachialis tendon
- Biceps (short head)
- Superior glenohumeral ligament
- Middle glenohumeral ligament
- Inferior glenohumeral ligament
- Triceps brachii (long head)

Coracoclavicular ligament
- Conoid ligament
- Trapezoid ligament

- Coracoacromial ligament

- Acromioclavicular ligament

- Joint capsule

- Acromion process
- Subacromial bursa
- Supraspinatus tendon (cut)
- Coracohumeral ligament
- Transverse humeral ligament
- Tendon sheath on tendon of long head of biceps brachi
- Subscapularis (cut)
- Biceps brachii (long head) tendon
- Humerus

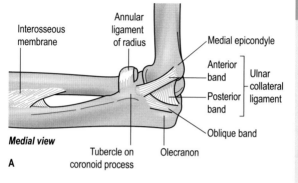

Medial view

A

Interosseous membrane

Annular ligament of radius

Medial epicondyle

Anterior band
Posterior band

Ulnar collateral ligament

Oblique band

Olecranon

Tubercle on coronoid process

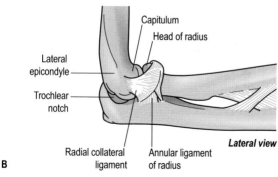

Lateral view

B

Capitulum
Head of radius

Lateral epicondyle

Trochlear notch

Radial collateral ligament

Annular ligament of radius

Figure 1.20 Ligaments of the elbow joint. **A** Medial. **B** Lateral.

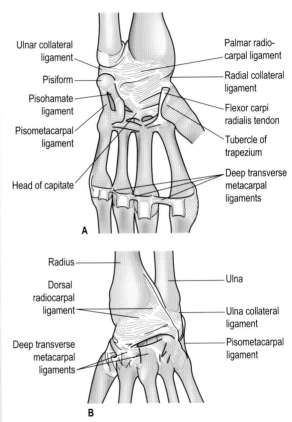

Ulnar collateral ligament

Pisiform

Pisohamate ligament

Pisometacarpal ligament

Head of capitate

Palmar radio-carpal ligament

Radial collateral ligament

Flexor carpi radialis tendon

Tubercle of trapezium

Deep transverse metacarpal ligaments

A

Radius

Dorsal radiocarpal ligament

Deep transverse metacarpal ligaments

Ulna

Ulna collateral ligament

Pisometacarpal ligament

B

Figure 1.21 Ligaments of the wrist and hand joints. **A** Anterior. **B** Posterior.

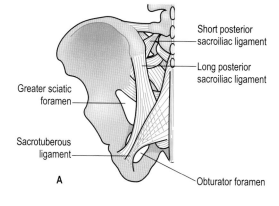

Short posterior sacroiliac ligament

Long posterior sacroiliac ligament

Greater sciatic foramen

Sacrotuberous ligament

Obturator foramen

A

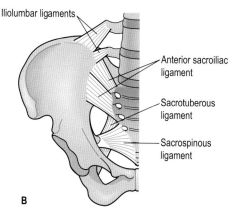

Iliolumbar ligaments

Anterior sacroiliac ligament

Sacrotuberous ligament

Sacrospinous ligament

B

Figure 1.22 Ligaments of the sacroiliac joint. **A** Posterior. **B** Anterior.

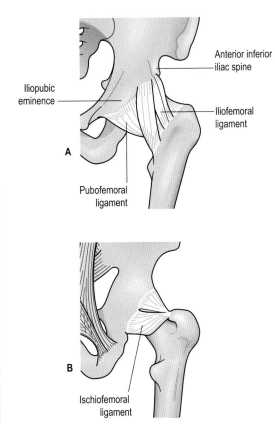

Figure 1.23 Ligaments of the hip joint. **A** Anterior. **B** Posterior.

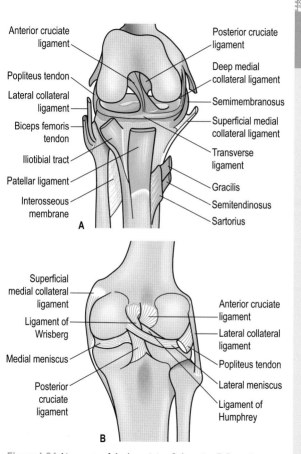

Figure 1.24 Ligaments of the knee joint. **A** Anterior. **B** Posterior.

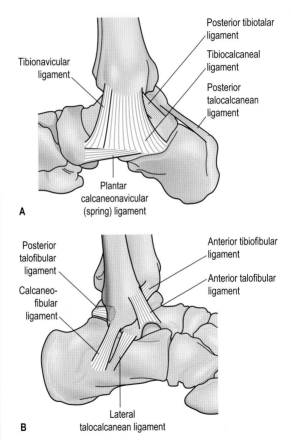

Figure 1.25 Ligaments of the ankle joint. **A** Medial. **B** Lateral.

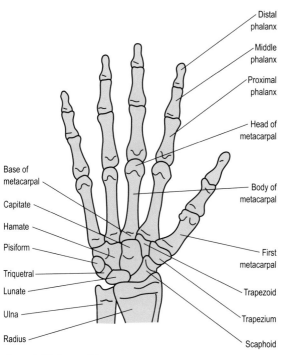

Distal
phalanx

Middle
phalanx

Proximal
phalanx

Head of
metacarpal

Base of
metacarpal

Capitate

Hamate

Pisiform

Triquetral

Lunate

Ulna

Radius

Body of
metacarpal

First
metacarpal

Trapezoid

Trapezium

Scaphoid

Figure 1.26 Bones of the right hand.

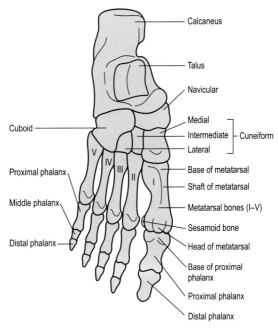

Calcaneus

Talus

Navicular

Medial
Intermediate ⎤ Cuneiform
Lateral

Cuboid

Base of metatarsal

Shaft of metatarsal

Proximal phalanx

Metatarsal bones (I–V)

Middle phalanx

Sesamoid bone

Head of metatarsal

Distal phalanx

Base of proximal
phalanx

Proximal phalanx

Distal phalanx

Figure 1.27 Bones of the right foot.

Nerve pathways

Brachial plexus

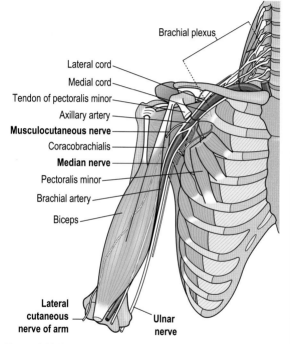

Brachial plexus

Lateral cord

Medial cord

Tendon of pectoralis minor

Axillary artery

Musculocutaneous nerve

Coracobrachialis

Median nerve

Pectoralis minor

Brachial artery

Biceps

Lateral cutaneous nerve of arm

Ulnar nerve

Figure 1.28 Brachial plexus.

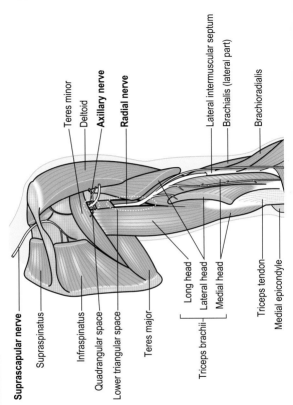

Teres minor
Deltoid
Axillary nerve
Radial nerve

Lateral intermuscular septum
Brachialis (lateral part)
Brachioradialis

Suprascapular nerve
Supraspinatus
Infraspinatus
Quadrangular space
Lower triangular space
Teres major

Long head
Lateral head
Medial head

Triceps brachii

Triceps tendon
Medial epicondyle

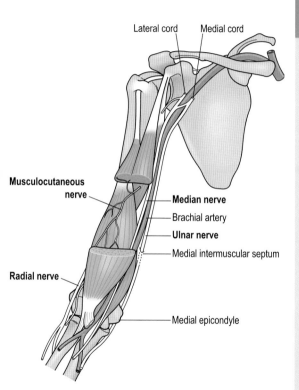

Lateral cord   Medial cord

**Musculocutaneous
nerve**

Median nerve

Brachial artery

Ulnar nerve

Medial intermuscular septum

Radial nerve

Medial epicondyle

Figure 1.30 Musculocutaneous, median and ulnar nerves.

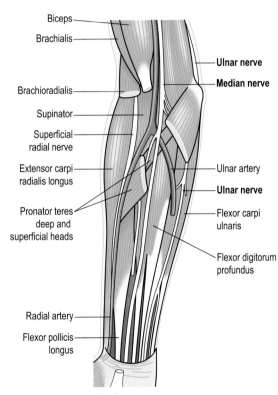

Biceps

Brachialis

Ulnar nerve

Median nerve

Brachioradialis

Supinator

Superficial
radial nerve

Extensor carpi
radialis longus

Ulnar artery

Ulnar nerve

Pronator teres
deep and
superficial heads

Flexor carpi
ulnaris

Flexor digitorum
profundus

Radial artery

Flexor pollicis
longus

Figure 1.31 Ulnar and median nerves.

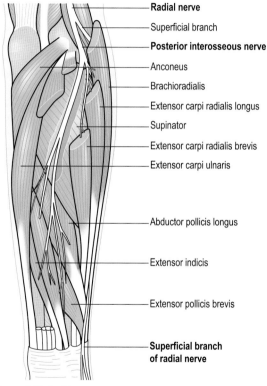

Radial nerve

Superficial branch

Posterior interosseous nerve

Anconeus

Brachioradialis

Extensor carpi radialis longus

Supinator

Extensor carpi radialis brevis

Extensor carpi ulnaris

Abductor pollicis longus

Extensor indicis

Extensor pollicis brevis

**Superficial branch
of radial nerve**

Figure 1.32 Radial nerve.

Lumbosacral plexus

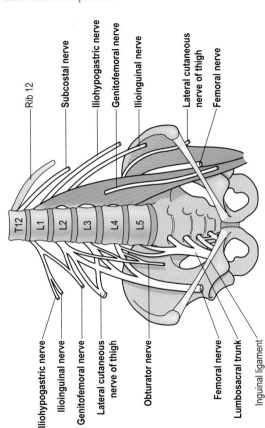

Figure 1.33 Lumbosacral plexus.

Rib 12
Subcostal nerve
Iliohypogastric nerve
Genitofemoral nerve
Ilioinguinal nerve
Lateral cutaneous nerve of thigh
Femoral nerve

T12
L1
L2
L3
L4
L5

Iliohypogastric nerve
Ilioinguinal nerve
Genitofemoral nerve
Lateral cutaneous nerve of thigh
Obturator nerve
Femoral nerve
Lumbosacral trunk
Inguinal ligament

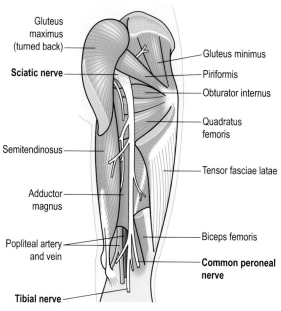

Gluteus maximus (turned back)

Sciatic nerve

Semitendinosus

Adductor magnus

Popliteal artery and vein

Tibial nerve

Gluteus minimus

Piriformis

Obturator internus

Quadratus femoris

Tensor fasciae latae

Biceps femoris

Common peroneal nerve

Figure 1.34 Sciatic nerve.

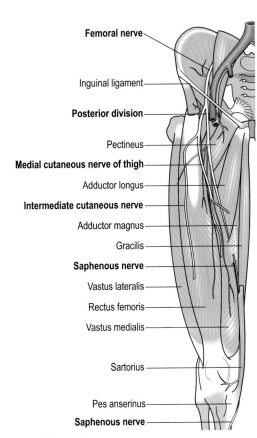

Femoral nerve

Inguinal ligament

Posterior division

Pectineus

Medial cutaneous nerve of thigh

Adductor longus

Intermediate cutaneous nerve

Adductor magnus

Gracilis

Saphenous nerve

Vastus lateralis

Rectus femoris

Vastus medialis

Sartorius

Pes anserinus

Saphenous nerve

Figure 1.35 Femoral nerve.

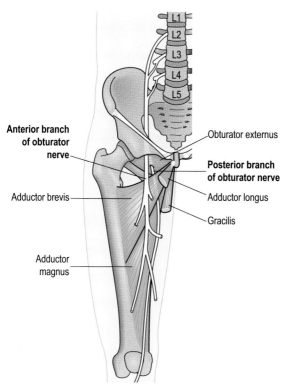

Anterior branch of obturator nerve

Obturator externus

Posterior branch of obturator nerve

Adductor brevis

Adductor longus

Gracilis

Adductor magnus

Figure 1.36 Obturator nerve.

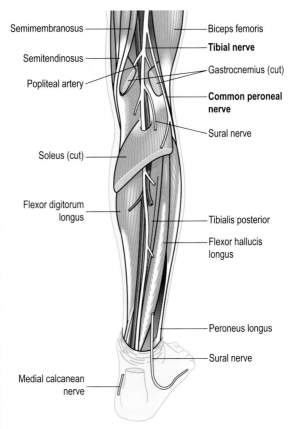

Semimembranosus

Semitendinosus

Popliteal artery

Soleus (cut)

Flexor digitorum
longus

Medial calcanean
nerve

Biceps femoris

Tibial nerve

Gastrocnemius (cut)

**Common peroneal
nerve**

Sural nerve

Tibialis posterior

Flexor hallucis
longus

Peroneus longus

Sural nerve

Figure 1.37 Tibial and common peroneal nerves.

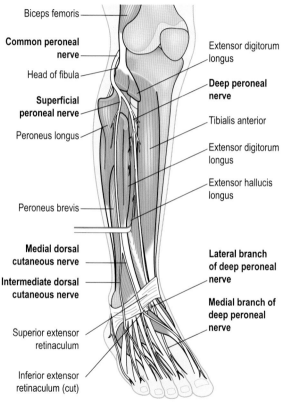

Figure 1.38 Superficial and deep peroneal nerves.

Axillary

Origin: Posterior cord (C5–C6)
Course:

- Descends laterally posterior to axillary artery and anterior to subscapularis
- Passes posteriorly at lower border of subscapularis together with posterior circumflex humeral vessels via quadrangular space
- Divides: anterior and posterior branches. Anterior branch winds around surgical neck of humerus and supplies anterior deltoid. Posterior branch supplies teres minor and posterior deltoid. Continues as upper lateral cutaneous nerve of the arm after passing around deltoid.

Musculocutaneous nerve

Origin: Large terminal branch of lateral cord (C5–C7)
Course:

- Descends from lower border of pectoralis minor, lateral to axillary artery
- Pierces coracobrachialis and descends diagonally between biceps and brachialis to lateral side of arm
- Pierces deep fascia of antecubital fossa and continues as lateral cutaneous nerve of the forearm
- Divides: anterior and posterior branches

Ulnar nerve

Origin: Large terminal branch of the medial cord (C7, C8, T1)
Course:

- Descends medial to brachial artery and anterior to triceps as far as the insertion of coracobrachialis
- Penetrates medial intermuscular septum and enters posterior compartment to continue descent anterior to medial head of triceps
- Passes posterior to medial epicondyle
- Enters anterior compartment between humeral and ulnar heads of flexor carpi ulnaris

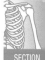

- Descends medially, anterior to flexor digitorum profundus and posterior to flexor carpi ulnaris
- Pierces deep fascia lateral to flexor carpi ulnaris and proximal to flexor retinaculum
- Passes anterior to flexor retinaculum and lateral to pisiform
- Crosses hook of hamate
- Divides: superficial and deep branches

Median nerve

Origin: Lateral cord (C5–C7) and medial cord (C8, T1)
Course:

- The two cords unite anterior to the third part of the axillary artery at the inferior margin of teres major
- Descends lateral to brachial artery and posterior to biceps passing medial and anterior to brachial artery at the insertion of coracobrachialis
- Crosses front of elbow lying on brachialis and deep to bicipital aponeurosis
- Dives between the two heads of pronator teres and descends through flexor digitorum superficialis and profundus
- Becomes superficial near the wrist passing between the tendons of flexor carpi radialis (lateral) and flexor digitorum superficialis (medial), deep to palmaris longus
- Passes through the carpal tunnel
- Divides: medial and lateral branches

Radial nerve

Origin: Posterior cord (C5–C8, T1)
Course:

- Descends posterior to axillary and brachial arteries and anterior to tendons of subscapularis, latissimus dorsi and teres major
- Enters posterior compartment via lower triangular space together with profunda brachii artery
- Descends obliquely towards lateral humerus along spiral groove lying between lateral and medial head of triceps

- Enters anterior compartment via lateral intermuscular septum to lie between brachialis and brachioradialis
- Divides: superficial radial nerve (sensory) and posterior interosseous nerve (motor) anterior to lateral epicondyle

Posterior interosseous nerve

Course:

- Enters posterior compartment between two heads of supinator
- Descends between deep and superficial groups of extensors
- Ends in flattened expansion on interosseous membrane

Sciatic nerve

Origin: Ventral rami (L4–S3)
Course:

- Forms anterior to piriformis. Leaves pelvis via greater sciatic foramen below piriformis
- Enters gluteal region approximately midway between ischial tuberosity and greater trochanter
- Descends on top of superior gemellus, obturator internus, inferior gemellus, quadratus femoris and adductor magnus and under gluteus maximus and long head of biceps femoris
- Divides: tibial and common peroneal nerves at approximately distal third of thigh

Tibial nerve

Origin: Medial terminal branch of sciatic nerve (L4–S3)
Course:

- Descends through popliteal fossa, passing laterally to medially across the popliteal vessels
- Passes under tendinous arch of soleus
- Descends inferomedially under soleus and gastrocnemius, lying on tibialis posterior and between flexor digitorum longus and flexor hallucis longus

- Passes through tarsal tunnel (formed by the flexor retinaculum, which extends from the medial malleolus to the medial calcaneus)
- Enters plantar aspect of foot
- Divides: medial and lateral plantar nerves

Common peroneal nerve

Origin: Lateral terminal branch of sciatic nerve (L4–S3)
Course:

- Descends along lateral side of popliteal fossa between biceps femoris and lateral head of gastrocnemius
- Passes anteriorly by winding around the neck of the fibula, deep to peroneus longus
- Divides: superficial and deep peroneal nerves

Superficial peroneal nerve

Course:

- Descends between extensor digitorum longus and peroneus longus, anterior to the fibula
- Pierces deep fascia halfway down the leg to become superficial
- Divides: medial and intermediate dorsal cutaneous nerves that enter foot via anterolateral aspect of ankle

Deep peroneal nerve

Course:

- Passes inferomedially into anterior compartment deep to extensor digitorum longus
- Descends on interosseous membrane deep to extensor hallucis longus and superior extensor retinaculum
- Crosses ankle deep to inferior extensor retinaculum and tendon of extensor hallucis longus and medial to tibialis anterior
- Enters dorsum of foot between tendons of extensor hallucis and digitorum longus
- Divides: medial and lateral branches

Obturator nerve

Origin: Anterior divisions of L2–L4
Course:

- Anterior divisions unite in psoas major
- Emerges from psoas major on lateral aspect of sacrum
- Crosses sacroiliac joint and obturator internus
- Enters obturator canal below superior pubic rami
- Exits obturator canal above obturator externus in medial compartment of thigh
- Divides: anterior and posterior branches (separated by obturator externus and adductor brevis)

Femoral nerve

Origin: Posterior divisions of L2–L4
Course:

- Posterior divisions unite in psoas major
- Emerges from lower lateral border of psoas major
- Descends in groove between psoas major and iliacus, deep to iliac fossa
- Passes posterior to inguinal ligament and lateral to femoral artery
- Enters femoral triangle
- Divides: number of anterior and posterior branches

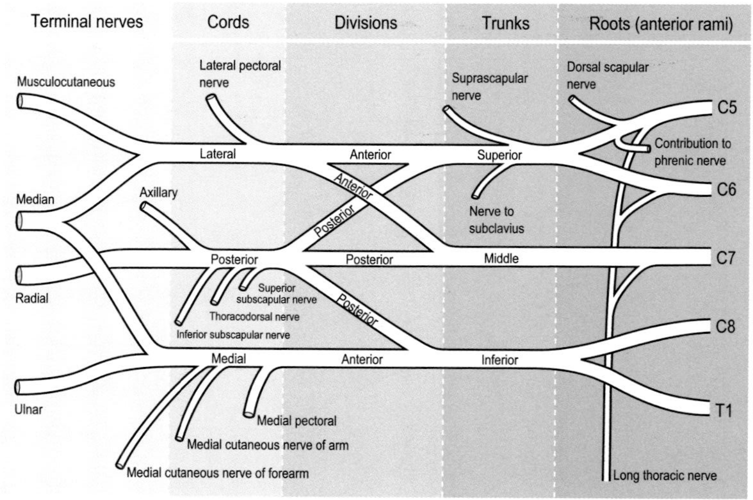

Brachial plexus

Roots (anterior rami)	Trunks	Divisions	Cords	Terminal nerves
C5				
Dorsal scapular nerve				
Contribution to phrenic nerve	Suprascapular nerve		Lateral pectoral nerve	Musculocutaneous
C6	Superior	Anterior	Lateral	
	Nerve to subclavius	Anterior		Axillary
C7	Middle	Posterior	Posterior	Median
		Posterior	Superior subscapular nerve	Radial
			Thoracodorsal nerve	
			Inferior subscapular nerve	
C8	Inferior	Anterior	Medial	
			Medial pectoral nerve	
			Medial cutaneous nerve of arm	Ulnar
T1			Medial cutaneous nerve of forearm	
Long thoracic nerve				

Figure I.39 Schematic of brachial plexus.

Lumbosacral plexus

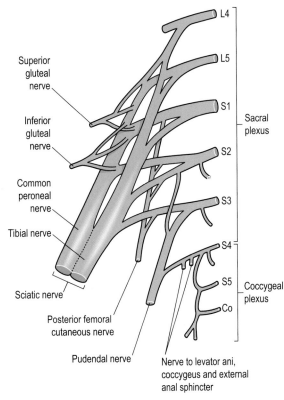

Figure 1.40 Schematic of lumbosacral plexus.

Peripheral nerve motor innervation (from O'Brien 2010, with permission)

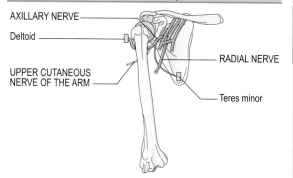

AXILLARY NERVE

Deltoid

UPPER CUTANEOUS NERVE OF THE ARM

RADIAL NERVE

Teres minor

Figure 1.41 Axillary nerve. (From O'Brien 2010, Aids to the Examination of the Peripheral Nervous System, 5e, with permission.)

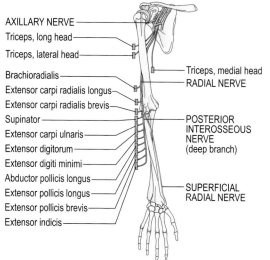

AXILLARY NERVE
Triceps, long head
Triceps, lateral head

Brachioradialis
Extensor carpi radialis longus
Extensor carpi radialis brevis
Supinator
Extensor carpi ulnaris
Extensor digitorum
Extensor digiti minimi
Abductor pollicis longus
Extensor pollicis longus
Extensor pollicis brevis
Extensor indicis

Triceps, medial head
RADIAL NERVE

POSTERIOR INTEROSSEOUS NERVE (deep branch)

SUPERFICIAL RADIAL NERVE

Figure 1.42 Radial nerve. (From O'Brien 2010, Aids to the Examination of the Peripheral Nervous System, 5e, with permission.)

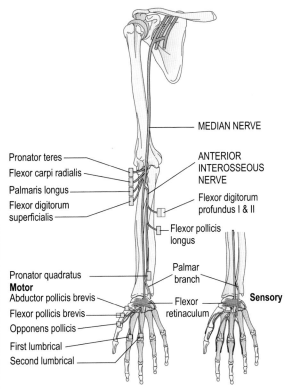

MEDIAN NERVE

Pronator teres

Flexor carpi radialis

Palmaris longus

Flexor digitorum
superficialis

ANTERIOR
INTEROSSEOUS
NERVE

Flexor digitorum
profundus I & II

Flexor pollicis
longus

Pronator quadratus
Motor
Abductor pollicis brevis

Flexor pollicis brevis

Opponens pollicis

First lumbrical

Second lumbrical

Palmar
branch

Flexor
retinaculum

Sensory

Figure 1.43 Median nerve. (From O'Brien 2010, Aids to the Examination of the Peripheral Nervous System, 5e, with permission.)

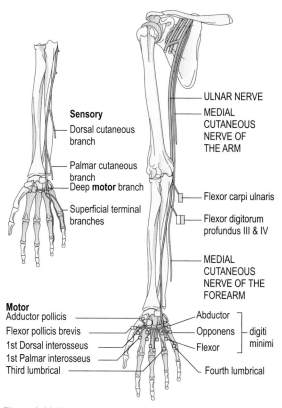

Sensory

- Dorsal cutaneous branch
- Palmar cutaneous branch
- Deep **motor** branch
- Superficial terminal branches

ULNAR NERVE

MEDIAL CUTANEOUS NERVE OF THE ARM

Flexor carpi ulnaris

Flexor digitorum profundus III & IV

MEDIAL CUTANEOUS NERVE OF THE FOREARM

Motor
- Adductor pollicis
- Flexor pollicis brevis
- 1st Dorsal interosseus
- 1st Palmar interosseus
- Third lumbrical

Abductor ⎤
Opponens ⎬ digiti minimi
Flexor ⎦

Fourth lumbrical

Figure 1.44 Ulnar nerve. (From O'Brien 2010, Aids to the Examination of the Peripheral Nervous System, 5e, with permission.)

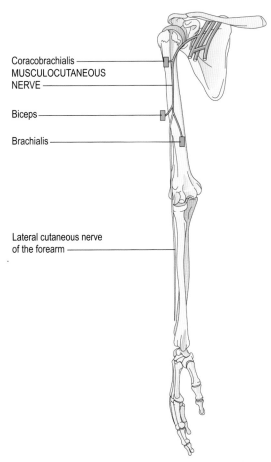

Coracobrachialis
MUSCULOCUTANEOUS
NERVE

Biceps

Brachialis

Lateral cutaneous nerve
of the forearm

Figure 1.45 Musculocutaneous nerve. (From O'Brien 2010, Aids to the Examination of the Peripheral Nervous System, 5e, with permission.)

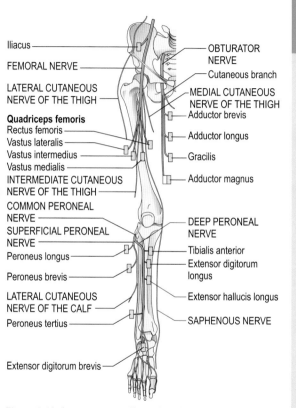

Iliacus

FEMORAL NERVE

LATERAL CUTANEOUS
NERVE OF THE THIGH

Quadriceps femoris
Rectus femoris
Vastus lateralis
Vastus intermedius
Vastus medialis
INTERMEDIATE CUTANEOUS
NERVE OF THE THIGH

COMMON PERONEAL
NERVE
SUPERFICIAL PERONEAL
NERVE
Peroneus longus

Peroneus brevis

LATERAL CUTANEOUS
NERVE OF THE CALF
Peroneus tertius

Extensor digitorum brevis

OBTURATOR
NERVE
Cutaneous branch

MEDIAL CUTANEOUS
NERVE OF THE THIGH
Adductor brevis

Adductor longus

Gracilis

Adductor magnus

DEEP PERONEAL
NERVE
Tibialis anterior
Extensor digitorum
longus

Extensor hallucis longus

SAPHENOUS NERVE

Figure 1.46 Anterior aspect of lower limb. (From O'Brien 2010,
Aids to the Examination of the Peripheral Nervous System, 5e, with
permission.)

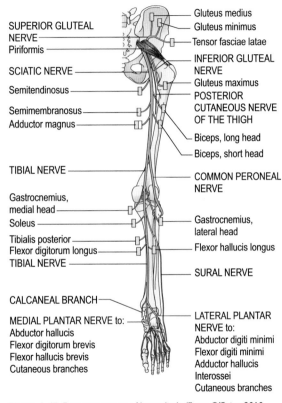

SUPERIOR GLUTEAL NERVE
Piriformis

SCIATIC NERVE

Semitendinosus

Semimembranosus
Adductor magnus

TIBIAL NERVE

Gastrocnemius, medial head

Soleus

Tibialis posterior
Flexor digitorum longus
TIBIAL NERVE

CALCANEAL BRANCH

MEDIAL PLANTAR NERVE to:
Abductor hallucis
Flexor digitorum brevis
Flexor hallucis brevis
Cutaneous branches

Gluteus medius
Gluteus minimus
Tensor fasciae latae
INFERIOR GLUTEAL NERVE
Gluteus maximus
POSTERIOR CUTANEOUS NERVE OF THE THIGH
Biceps, long head
Biceps, short head

COMMON PERONEAL NERVE

Gastrocnemius, lateral head

Flexor hallucis longus

SURAL NERVE

LATERAL PLANTAR NERVE to:
Abductor digiti minimi
Flexor digiti minimi
Adductor hallucis
Interossei
Cutaneous branches

Figure 1.47 Posterior aspect of lower limb. (From O'Brien 2010, Aids to the Examination of the Peripheral Nervous System, 5e, with permission.)

Muscle innervation chart (data from Standring 2015, with permission)

Upper limb

C1	C2	C3	C4	C5	C6	C7	C8	T1
Inferior and superior oblique								
Rectus capitis posterior major and minor								
Rectus capitis anterior and lateralis								
Longus capitis								
	Longissimus cervicis							
	Longus colli							
		Levator scapulae						
		Trapezius						
		Diaphragm						
		Splenius capitis						
		Scalenus medius						
			Rhomboid major					
			Rhomboid minor					
			Scalenus anterior					
			Longissimus capitis					
				Biceps brachii				
				Brachioradialis				

C1	C2	C3	C4	C5	C6	C7	C8	T1
				Deltoid				
				Infraspinatus				
				Subscapularis				
				Supraspinatus				
				Teres minor				
				Brachialis				
					Coracobrachialis			
				Serratus anterior				
				Splenius cervicis				
				Teres major				
				Pectoralis major				
				Pectoralis minor				
					Extensor carpi radialis longus			
					Flexor carpi radialis			
					Pronator teres			
					Supinator			
					Anconeus			
					Latissimus dorsi			
					Scalenus posterior			
					Triceps brachii			
						Abductor pollicis longus		
						Extensor carpi radialis brevis		
						Extensor carpi ulnaris		

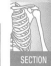

C1	C2	C3	C4	C5	C6	C7	C8	T1
						Extensor digiti minimi		
						Extensor digitorum		
						Extensor indicis		
						Extensor pollicis brevis		
						Extensor pollicis longus		
						Flexor pollicis longus		
						Palmaris longus		
						Pronator quadratus		
						Flexor carpi ulnaris		
							Abductor digiti minimi	
							Abductor pollicis brevis	
							Adductor pollicis	
							Dorsal interossei	
							Flexor digiti minimi brevis	
							Flexor digitorum profundus	

C1	C2	C3	C4	C5	C6	C7	C8	T1
								Flexor digitorum superficialis
								Flexor pollicis brevis
								Lumbricals
								Opponens digiti minimi
								Opponens pollicis
								Palmar interossei

Lower limb

T12	L1	L2	L3	L4	L5	S1	S2	S3
Quadratus lumborum								
	Psoas minor							
	Psoas major							
		Adductor brevis						
		Gracilis						
		Iliacus						
		Pectineus						
		Sartorius						
		Adductor longus						
		Adductor magnus						
		Rectus femoris						

T12	L1	L2	L3	L4	L5	S1	S2	S3
		Vastus intermedius						
		Vastus lateralis						
		Vastus medialis						
			Obturator externus					
			Gluteus medius					
			Gluteus minimus					
			Popliteus					
				Tibialis anterior				
				Tibialis posterior				
				Tensor fascia lata				
					Extensor hallucis longus			
					Extensor digitorum brevis			
					Extensor digitorum longus			
					Gemellus inferior			
					Gemellus superior			
					Obturator internus			
					Peroneus brevis			
					Peroneus longus			
					Peroneus tertius			
					Quadratus femoris			

NEUROMUSCULOSKELETAL ANATOMY

T12	L1	L2	L3	L4	L5	S1	S2	S3
					Biceps femoris			
					Flexor digitorum longus			
					Flexor hallucis longus			
					Gluteus maximus			
					Piriformis			
					Semimembranosus			
					Semitendinosus			
						Abductor hallucis		
						Flexor digitorum brevis		
						Flexor hallucis brevis		
						Gastrocnemius		
						Plantaris		
						Soleus		
						Abductor digiti minimi		
						Flexor digitorum accessorius		
							Adductor hallucis	
							Dorsal interossei	
							Flexor digiti minimi brevis	
							Lumbricals	
							Plantar interossei	

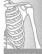
Muscles listed by function

Head and neck

Flexors: longus colli, longus capitis, rectus capitis anterior, sternocleidomastoid, scalenus anterior

Lateral flexors: erector spinae, rectus capitis lateralis, scalenes (anterior, medius and posterior), splenius cervicis, splenius capitis, trapezius, levator scapulae, sternocleidomastoid

Extensors: levator scapulae, splenius cervicis, trapezius, splenius capitis, semispinalis, superior oblique, sternocleidomastoid, erector spinae, rectus capitis posterior major, rectus capitis posterior minor

Rotators: semispinalis, multifidus, scalenus anterior, splenius cervicis, sternocleidomastoid, splenius capitis, rectus capitis posterior major, inferior oblique

Trunk

Flexors: rectus abdominis, external oblique, internal oblique, psoas minor, psoas major, iliacus

Rotators: multifidus, rotatores, semispinalis, internal oblique, external oblique

Lateral flexors: quadratus lumborum, intertransversarii, external oblique, internal oblique, erector spinae, multifidus

Extensors: quadratus lumborum, multifidus, semispinalis, erector spinae, interspinales, rotatores

Scapula

Retractors: rhomboid minor, rhomboid major, trapezius, levator scapulae

Protractors: serratus anterior, pectoralis minor

Elevators: trapezius, levator scapulae

Depressors: trapezius

Lateral rotators: trapezius, serratus anterior

Medial rotators: rhomboid major, rhomboid minor, pectoralis minor, levator scapulae

Shoulder

Flexors: pectoralis major, deltoid (anterior fibres), biceps brachii (long head), coracobrachialis

59

Extensors: latissimus dorsi, teres major, pectoralis major, deltoid (posterior fibres), triceps (long head)

Abductors: supraspinatus, deltoid (middle fibres)

Adductors: coracobrachialis, pectoralis major, latissimus dorsi, teres major

Medial rotators: subscapularis, teres major, latissimus dorsi, pectoralis major, deltoid (anterior fibres)

Lateral rotators: teres minor, infraspinatus, deltoid (posterior fibres)

Elbow

Flexors: biceps brachii, brachialis, brachioradialis, pronator teres

Extensors: triceps brachii, anconeus

Pronators: pronator teres, pronator quadratus

Supinators: supinator, biceps brachii

Wrist

Flexors: flexor carpi ulnaris, flexor carpi radialis, palmaris longus, flexor digitorum superficialis, flexor digitorum profundus, flexor pollicis longus

Extensors: extensor carpi radialis longus, extensor carpi radialis brevis, extensor carpi ulnaris, extensor digitorum, extensor indicis, extensor digiti minimi, extensor pollicis longus, extensor pollicis brevis

Ulnar deviation: flexor carpi ulnaris, extensor carpi ulnaris

Radial deviation: flexor carpi radialis, extensor carpi radialis longus, extensor carpi radialis brevis, abductor pollicis longus, extensor pollicis longus, extensor pollicis brevis

Fingers

Flexors: flexor digitorum superficialis, flexor digitorum profundus, lumbricals, flexor digiti minimi brevis

Extensors: extensor digitorum, extensor digiti minimi, extensor indicis, interossei, lumbricals

Abductors: dorsal interossei, abductor digiti minimi, opponens digiti minimi

Adductors: palmar interossei

Thumb

Flexors: flexor pollicis longus, flexor pollicis brevis
Extensors: extensor pollicis longus, extensor pollicis brevis, abductor pollicis longus
Abductors: abductor pollicis longus, abductor pollicis brevis
Adductors: adductor pollicis
Opposition: opponens pollicis

Hip

Flexors: psoas major, iliacus, rectus femoris, sartorius, pectineus
Extensors: gluteus maximus, semitendinosus, semimembranosus, biceps femoris
Abductors: gluteus maximus, gluteus medius, gluteus minimus, tensor fascia lata, sartorius, piriformis
Adductors: adductor magnus, adductor longus, adductor brevis, gracilis, pectineus
Medial rotators: gluteus medius, gluteus minimus, tensor fascia lata
Lateral rotators: gluteus maximus, piriformis, obturator internus, gemellus superior, gemellus inferior, quadratus femoris, obturator externus, sartorius

Knee

Flexors: semitendinosus, semimembranosus, biceps femoris, gastrocnemius, gracilis, sartorius, plantaris, popliteus
Extensors: rectus femoris, vastus lateralis, vastus intermedius, vastus medialis, tensor fascia lata
Tibial lateral rotators: biceps femoris
Tibial medial rotators: semitendinosus, semimembranosus, gracilis, sartorius, popliteus

Ankle

Plantarflexors: gastrocnemius, soleus, plantaris, peroneus longus, tibialis posterior, flexor digitorum longus, flexor hallucis longus, peroneus brevis
Dorsiflexors: tibialis anterior, extensor digitorum longus, extensor hallucis longus, peroneus tertius
Invertors: tibialis anterior, tibialis posterior
Evertors: peroneus longus, peroneus tertius, peroneus brevis

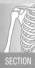
Toes

Flexors: flexor digitorum longus, flexor digitorum accessorius, flexor digitorum brevis, flexor hallucis longus, flexor hallucis brevis, flexor digiti minimi brevis, interossei, lumbricals, abductor hallucis

Extensors: extensor hallucis longus, extensor digitorum longus, extensor digitorum brevis, lumbricals, interossei

Abductors: abductor hallucis, abductor digiti minimi, dorsal interossei

Adductors: adductor hallucis, plantar interossei

Alphabetical listing of muscles

Abductor digiti minimi (foot)

Action: abducts fifth toe
Origin: calcaneal tuberosity, plantar aponeurosis, intermuscular septum
Insertion: lateral side of base of proximal phalanx of fifth toe
Nerve: lateral plantar nerve (S1–S3)

Abductor digiti minimi (hand)

Action: abducts little finger
Origin: pisiform, tendon of flexor carpi ulnaris, pisohamate ligament
Insertion: ulnar side of base of proximal phalanx of little finger
Nerve: ulnar nerve (C8, T1)

Abductor hallucis

Action: abducts and flexes great toe
Origin: flexor retinaculum, calcaneal tuberosity, plantar aponeurosis, intermuscular septum
Insertion: medial side of base of proximal phalanx of great toe
Nerve: medial plantar nerve (S1, S2)

Abductor pollicis brevis

Action: abducts thumb

Origin: flexor retinaculum, tubercles of scaphoid and trapezium, tendon of abductor pollicis longus
Insertion: radial side of base of proximal phalanx of thumb
Nerve: median nerve (C8, T1)

Abductor pollicis longus

Action: abducts and extends thumb, abducts wrist
Origin: upper part of posterior surface of ulna, middle third of posterior surface of radius, interosseous membrane
Insertion: radial side of first metacarpal base, trapezium
Nerve: posterior interosseous nerve (C7, C8)

Adductor brevis

Action: adducts hip
Origin: external aspect of body and inferior ramus of pubis
Insertion: upper half of linea aspera
Nerve: obturator nerve (L2, L3)

Adductor hallucis

Action: adducts great toe
Origin: oblique head – bases of second to fourth metatarsal, sheath of peroneus longus tendon; transverse head – plantar metatarsophalangeal ligaments of lateral three toes
Insertion: lateral side of base of proximal phalanx of great toe
Nerve: lateral plantar nerve (S2, S3)

Adductor longus

Action: adducts thigh
Origin: front of pubis
Insertion: middle third of linea aspera
Nerve: anterior division of obturator nerve (L2–L4)

Adductor magnus

Action: adducts thigh
Origin: inferior ramus of pubis, conjoined ischial ramus, inferolateral aspect of ischial tuberosity
Insertion: linea aspera, proximal part of medial supracondylar line

Nerve: obturator nerve and tibial division of sciatic nerve
(L2–L4)

Adductor pollicis

Action: adducts thumb
Origin: oblique head – palmar ligaments of carpus, flexor
carpi radialis tendon, base of second to fourth
metacarpals, capitate; transverse head – palmar surface of
third metacarpal
Insertion: base of proximal phalanx of thumb
Nerve: ulnar nerve (C8, T1)

Anconeus

Action: extends elbow
Origin: posterior surface of lateral epicondyle of humerus
Insertion: lateral surface of olecranon, upper quarter of
posterior surface of ulna
Nerve: radial nerve (C6–C8)

Biceps brachii

Action: flexes shoulder and elbow, supinates forearm
Origin: long head – supraglenoid tubercle of scapula and
glenoid labrum; short head – apex of coracoid process
Insertion: posterior part of radial tuberosity, bicipital
aponeurosis into deep fascia over common flexor
origin
Nerve: musculocutaneous nerve (C5, C6)

Biceps femoris

Action: flexes knee and extends hip, laterally rotates tibia on
femur
Origin: long head – ischial tuberosity, sacrotuberous ligament;
short head – lower half of lateral lip of linea aspera,
lateral supracondylar line of femur, lateral intermuscular
septum
Insertion: head of fibula, lateral tibial condyle
Nerve: sciatic nerve (L5–S2). Long head – tibial division; short
head – common peroneal division

Brachialis

Action: flexes elbow
Origin: lower half of anterior surface of humerus, intermuscular septum
Insertion: coronoid process and tuberosity of ulna
Nerve: musculocutaneous nerve (C5, C6), radial nerve (C7)

Brachioradialis

Action: flexes elbow
Origin: upper two-thirds of lateral supracondylar ridge of humerus, lateral intermuscular septum
Insertion: lateral side of radius above styloid process
Nerve: radial nerve (C5, C6)

Coracobrachialis

Action: adducts shoulder and acts as weak flexor
Origin: apex of coracoid process
Insertion: midway along medial border of humerus
Nerve: musculocutaneous nerve (C5–C7)

Deltoid

Action: anterior fibres – flex and medially rotate shoulder; middle fibres – abduct shoulder; posterior fibres – extend and laterally rotate shoulder
Origin: anterior fibres – anterior border of lateral third of clavicle; middle fibres – lateral margin of acromion process; posterior fibres – lower edge of crest of spine of scapula
Insertion: deltoid tuberosity of humerus
Nerve: axillary nerve (C5, C6)

Diaphragm

Action: draws central tendon inferiorly. Changes volume and pressure of thoracic and abdominal cavities
Origin: posterior surface of xiphoid process, lower six costal cartilages and adjoining ribs on each side, medial and lateral arcuate ligaments, anterolateral aspect of bodies of lumbar vertebrae

Insertion: central tendon
Nerve: phrenic nerves (C3–C5)

Dorsal interossei (foot)

Action: abducts toes, flexes metatarsophalangeal joints
Origin: proximal half of sides of adjacent metatarsals
Insertion: bases of proximal phalanges and dorsal digital
    expansion (first attaches medially to second toe; second,
    third and fourth attach laterally to second, third and
    fourth toes, respectively)
Nerve: lateral plantar nerve (S2, S3)

Dorsal interossei (hand)

Action: abducts index, middle and ring fingers, flexes
    metacarpophalangeal joints and extends interphalangeal
    joints
Origin: adjacent sides of two metacarpal bones (four
    bipennate muscles)
Insertion: bases of proximal phalanges and dorsal digital
    expansions (first attaches laterally to index finger; second
    and third attach to both sides of middle finger; fourth
    attaches medially to ring finger)
Nerve: ulnar nerve (C8, T1)

Erector spinae

See iliocostalis, longissimus and spinalis

Extensor carpi radialis brevis

Action: extends and abducts wrist
Origin: lateral epicondyle via common extensor tendon
Insertion: posterior surface of base of third metacarpal
Nerve: posterior interosseous branch of radial nerve (C7, C8)

Extensor carpi radialis longus

Action: extends and abducts wrist
Origin: lower third of lateral supracondylar ridge of humerus,
    intermuscular septa
Insertion: posterior surface of base of second metacarpal
Nerve: radial nerve (C6, C7)

Extensor carpi ulnaris

Action: extends and adducts wrist
Origin: lateral epicondyle via common extensor tendon
Insertion: medial side of fifth metacarpal base
Nerve: posterior interosseous nerve (C7, C8)

Extensor digiti minimi

Action: extends fifth digit and wrist
Origin: lateral epicondyle via common extensor tendon,
  intermuscular septa
Insertion: dorsal digital expansion of fifth digit
Nerve: posterior interosseous nerve (C7, C8)

Extensor digitorum

Action: extends fingers and wrist
Origin: lateral epicondyle via common extensor tendon,
  intermuscular septa
Insertion: lateral and dorsal surfaces of second to fifth digits
Nerve: posterior interosseous branch of radial nerve (C7, C8)

Extensor digitorum brevis

Action: extends great toe and adjacent three toes
Origin: superolateral surface of calcaneus, inferior extensor
  retinaculum, interosseous talocalcaneal ligament
Insertion: base of proximal phalanx of great toe, lateral side of
  dorsal hood of adjacent three toes
Nerve: deep peroneal nerve (L5, S1)

Extensor digitorum longus

Action: extends lateral four toes, ankle dorsiflexor
Origin: upper three-quarters of medial surface of fibula,
  interosseous membrane, lateral tibial condyle
Insertion: middle and distal phalanges of four lateral toes
Nerve: deep peroneal nerve (L5, S1)

Extensor hallucis longus

Action: extends great toe, ankle dorsiflexor
Origin: middle half of medial surface of fibula, interosseous
  membrane

Insertion: base of distal phalanx of great toe
Nerve: deep peroneal nerve (L5)

Extensor indicis

Action: extends index finger and wrist
Origin: lower part of posterior surface of ulna, interosseous
    membrane
Insertion: dorsal digital expansion on back of proximal
    phalanx of index finger
Nerve: posterior interosseous nerve (C7, C8)

Extensor pollicis brevis

Action: extends thumb and wrist, abducts wrist
Origin: posterior surface of radius, interosseous membrane
Insertion: dorsolateral base of proximal phalanx of
    thumb
Nerve: posterior interosseous nerve (C7, C8)

Extensor pollicis longus

Action: extends thumb and wrist, abducts wrist
Origin: middle third of posterior surface of ulna, interosseous
    membrane
Insertion: dorsal surface of distal phalanx of thumb
Nerve: posterior interosseous nerve (C7, C8)

External oblique

Action: flexes, laterally flexes and rotates trunk
Origin: outer borders of lower eight ribs and their costal
    cartilages
Insertion: outer lip of anterior two-thirds of iliac crest,
    abdominal aponeurosis to linea alba stretching from
    xiphoid process to symphysis pubis
Nerve: ventral rami of lower six thoracic nerves (T7–T12)

Flexor carpi radialis

Action: flexes and abducts wrist
Origin: medial epicondyle via common flexor tendon
Insertion: front of base of second and third
Nerve: median (C6, C7)

Flexor carpi ulnaris

Action: flexes and adducts wrist
Origin: humeral head – medial epicondyle via common flexor
tendon; ulnar head – medial border of olecranon and
upper two-thirds of border of ulna
Insertion: pisiform, hook of hamate and base of fifth
metacarpal
Nerve: ulnar nerve (C7–T1)

Flexor digiti minimi brevis (foot)

Action: flexes fifth metatarsophalangeal joint, supports lateral
longitudinal arch
Origin: plantar aspect of base of fifth metatarsal, sheath of
peroneus longus tendon
Insertion: lateral side of base of proximal phalanx of fifth
toe
Nerve: lateral plantar nerve (S2, S3)

Flexor digiti minimi brevis (hand)

Action: flexes little finger
Origin: hook of hamate, flexor retinaculum
Insertion: ulnar side of base of proximal phalanx of little
finger
Nerve: ulnar nerve (C8, T1)

Flexor digitorum accessorius

Action: flexes distal phalanges of lateral four toes
Origin: medial head – medial tubercle of calcaneus; lateral
head – lateral tubercle of calcaneus and long plantar
ligament
Insertion: flexor digitorum longus tendon
Nerve: lateral plantar nerve (S1–S3)

Flexor digitorum brevis

Action: flexes proximal interphalangeal joints and
metatarsophalangeal joints of lateral four toes
Origin: calcaneal tuberosity, plantar aponeurosis,
intermuscular septa

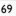

Insertion: tendons divide and attach to both sides of base of
    middle phalanges of second to fifth toes
Nerve: medial plantar nerve (S1, S2)

Flexor digitorum longus

Action: flexes lateral four toes, plantarflexes ankle
Origin: medial part of posterior surface of tibia, deep
    transverse fascia
Insertion: plantar aspect of base of distal phalanges of second
    to fifth toes
Nerve: tibial nerve (L5–S2)

Flexor digitorum profundus

Action: flexes fingers and wrist
Origin: medial side of coronoid process of ulna, upper
    three-quarters of anterior and medial surfaces of ulna,
    interosseous membrane
Insertion: base of palmar surface of distal phalanx of second
    to fifth digits
Nerve: medial part – ulnar nerve (C8, T1); lateral part –
    anterior interosseous branch of median nerve (C8, T1)

Flexor digitorum superficialis

Action: flexes fingers and wrist
Origin: humeroulnar head – medial epicondyle via common
    flexor tendon, medial part of coronoid process of ulna,
    ulnar collateral ligament, intermuscular septa; radial head
    – upper two-thirds of anterior border of radius
Insertion: tendons divide and insert into sides of shaft of
    middle phalanx of second to fifth digits
Nerve: median (C8, T1)

Flexor hallucis brevis

Action: flexes metatarsophalangeal joint of great toe
Origin: medial side of plantar surface of cuboid, lateral
    cuneiform
Insertion: medial and lateral side of base of proximal phalanx
    of great toe

Nerve: medial plantar nerve (S1, S2)

Flexor hallucis longus

Action: flexes great toe, plantarflexes ankle
Origin: lower two-thirds of posterior surface of fibula, interosseous membrane, intermuscular septum
Insertion: plantar surface of base of distal phalanx of great toe
Nerve: tibial nerve (L5–S2)

Flexor pollicis brevis

Action: flexes metacarpophalangeal joint of thumb
Origin: flexor retinaculum, tubercle of trapezium, capitate, trapezoid
Insertion: base of proximal phalanx of thumb
Nerve: median nerve (C8–T1). Sometimes also supplied by ulnar nerve (C8–T1)

Flexor pollicis longus

Action: flexes thumb and wrist
Origin: anterior surface of radius, interosseous membrane
Insertion: palmar surface of distal phalanx of thumb
Nerve: anterior interosseous branch of median nerve (C7, C8)

Gastrocnemius

Action: plantarflexes ankle, flexes knee
Origin: medial head – posterior part of medial femoral condyle; lateral head – lateral surface of lateral femoral condyle
Insertion: posterior surface of calcaneus
Nerve: tibial nerve (S1, S2)

Gemellus inferior

Action: laterally rotates hip
Origin: upper part of ischial tuberosity
Insertion: with obturator internus tendon into medial surface of greater trochanter
Nerve: nerve to quadratus femoris (L5, S1)

Gemellus superior

Action: laterally rotates hip
Origin: gluteal surface of ischial spine

Insertion: with obturator internus tendon into medial surface of greater trochanter

Nerve: nerve to obturator internus (L5, S1)

Gluteus maximus

Action: extends, laterally rotates and abducts hip

Origin: posterior gluteal line of ilium, posterior border of ilium and adjacent part of iliac crest, aponeurosis of erector spinae, posterior aspect of sacrum, side of coccyx, sacrotuberous ligament, gluteal aponeurosis

Insertion: iliotibial tract of fascia lata, gluteal tuberosity of femur

Nerve: inferior gluteal nerve (L5–S2)

Gluteus medius

Action: abducts and medially rotates hip

Origin: gluteal surface of ilium between posterior and anterior gluteal lines

Insertion: superolateral side of greater trochanter

Nerve: superior gluteal nerve (L4–S1)

Gluteus minimus

Action: abducts and medially rotates hip

Origin: gluteal surface of ilium between anterior and inferior gluteal lines

Insertion: anterolateral ridge on greater trochanter

Nerve: superior gluteal nerve (L4–S1)

Gracilis

Action: flexes knee, adducts hip, medially rotates tibia on femur

Origin: lower half of body and inferior ramus of pubis, adjacent ischial ramus

Insertion: upper part of medial surface of tibia

Nerve: obturator nerve (L2, L3)

Iliacus

Action: flexes hip and trunk

Origin: superior two-thirds of iliac fossa, inner lip of iliac crest, ala of sacrum, anterior sacroiliac and iliolumbar ligaments

Insertion: blends with insertion of psoas major into lesser trochanter
Nerve: femoral nerve (L2, L3)

Iliocostalis cervicis

Action: extends and laterally flexes vertebral column
Origin: angles of third to sixth ribs
Insertion: posterior tubercles of transverse processes of C4 to C6
Nerve: dorsal rami

Iliocostalis lumborum

Action: extends and laterally flexes vertebral column
Origin: medial and lateral sacral crests, spines of T11, T12 and lumbar vertebrae and their supraspinous ligaments, medial part of iliac crest
Insertion: angles of lower six or seven ribs
Nerve: dorsal rami

Iliocostalis thoracis

Action: extends and laterally flexes vertebral column
Origin: angles of lower six ribs
Insertion: angles of upper six ribs, transverse process of C7
Nerve: dorsal rami

Inferior oblique

Action: rotates atlas and head
Origin: lamina of axis
Insertion: transverse process of atlas
Nerve: dorsal ramus (C1)

Infraspinatus

Action: laterally rotates shoulder
Origin: medial two-thirds of infraspinous fossa and infraspinous fascia
Insertion: middle facet on greater tubercle of humerus, posterior aspect of capsule of shoulder joint
Nerve: suprascapular nerve (C5, C6)

Intercostales externi

Action: elevate rib below toward rib above to increase thoracic cavity volume for inspiration
Origin: lower border of rib above
Insertion: upper border of rib below
Nerve: intercostal nerves

Intercostales interni

Action: draw ribs downward to decrease thoracic cavity volume for expiration
Origin: lower border of costal cartilage and costal groove of rib above
Insertion: upper border of rib below
Nerve: intercostal nerves

Internal oblique

Action: flexes, laterally flexes and rotates trunk
Origin: lateral two-thirds of inguinal ligament, anterior two-thirds of intermediate line of iliac crest, thoracolumbar fascia
Insertion: lower four ribs and their cartilages, crest of pubis, abdominal aponeurosis to linea alba
Nerve: ventral rami of lower six thoracic nerves, first lumbar nerve

Interspinales

Action: extend and stabilize vertebral column
Origin and insertion: extend between adjacent spinous processes (best developed in cervical and lumbar regions – sometimes absent in thoracic)
Nerve: dorsal rami of spinal nerves

Intertransversarii

Action: laterally flex lumbar and cervical spine, stabilize vertebral column
Origin: transverse processes of cervical and lumbar vertebrae
Insertion: transverse process of vertebra superior to origin
Nerve: ventral and dorsal rami of spinal nerves

Latissimus dorsi

Action: extends, adducts and medially rotates shoulder
Origin: spinous processes of lower six thoracic and all
   lumbar and sacral vertebrae, intervening supra- and
   interspinous ligaments, outer lip of iliac crest, outer
   surfaces of lower three or four ribs, inferior angle of
   scapula
Insertion: intertubercular sulcus of humerus
Nerve: thoracodorsal nerve (C6–C8)

Levator scapulae

Action: elevates, medially rotates and retracts scapula, extends
   and laterally flexes neck
Origin: transverse processes of C1–C3/4
Insertion: medial border of scapula between superior angle
   and base of spine
Nerve: ventral rami (C3, C4), dorsal scapular nerve (C5)

Longissimus capitis

Action: extends, laterally flexes and rotates head
Origin: transverse processes of T1–T4/5, articular processes
   of C4/5–C7
Insertion: posterior aspect of mastoid process
Nerve: dorsal rami

Longissimus cervicis

Action: extends and laterally flexes vertebral column
Origin: transverse processes of T1–T4/5
Insertion: transverse processes of C2–C6
Nerve: dorsal rami

Longissimus thoracis

Action: extends and laterally flexes vertebral column
Origin: transverse and accessory processes of lumbar
   vertebrae and thoracolumbar fascia
Insertion: transverse processes of T1–T12 and lower nine or
   ten ribs
Nerve: dorsal rami

Longus capitis

Action: flexes neck
Origin: occipital bone
Insertion: anterior tubercles of transverse processes of C3–C6
Nerve: anterior primary rami (C1–C3)

Longus colli

Action: flexes neck
Origin: inferior oblique part – front of bodies of T1–T2/3; vertical intermediate part – front of bodies of T1–T3 and C5–C7; superior oblique part – anterior tubercles of transverse processes of C3–C5
Insertion: inferior oblique part – anterior tubercles of transverse processes of C5 and C6; vertical intermediate part – front of bodies of C2–C4; superior oblique part – anterior tubercle of atlas
Nerve: anterior primary rami (C2–C6)

Lumbricals (foot)

Action: flexes metatarsophalangeal joints and extends interphalangeal joints of lateral four toes
Origin: tendons of flexor digitorum longus
Insertion: medial side of extensor hood and base of proximal phalanx of lateral four toes
Nerve: first lumbrical – medial plantar nerve (S2, S3); lateral three lumbricals – lateral plantar nerve (S2, S3)

Lumbricals (hand)

Action: flexes metacarpophalangeal joints and extends interphalangeal joints of fingers
Origin: tendons of flexor digitorum profundus
Insertion: lateral margin of dorsal digital expansion of extensor digitorum
Nerve: first and second – median nerve (C8, T1); third and fourth – ulnar nerve (C8, T1)

Multifidus

Action: extends, rotates and laterally flexes vertebral column

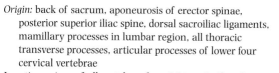
Origin: back of sacrum, aponeurosis of erector spinae, posterior superior iliac spine, dorsal sacroiliac ligaments, mamillary processes in lumbar region, all thoracic transverse processes, articular processes of lower four cervical vertebrae

Insertion: spines of all vertebrae from L5 to axis (deep layer attaches to vertebrae above; middle layer attaches to second or third vertebrae above; outer layer attaches to third or fourth vertebrae above)

Nerve: dorsal rami of spinal nerves

Obturator externus

Action: laterally rotates hip

Origin: outer surface of obturator membrane and adjacent bone of pubic and ischial rami

Insertion: trochanteric fossa of femur

Nerve: posterior branch of obturator nerve (L3, L4)

Obturator internus

Action: laterally rotates hip

Origin: internal surface of obturator membrane and surrounding bony margin

Insertion: medial surface of greater trochanter

Nerve: nerve to obturator internus (L5, S1)

Opponens digiti minimi

Action: abducts fifth digit, pulls it forward and rotates it laterally

Origin: hook of hamate, flexor retinaculum

Insertion: medial border of fifth metacarpal

Nerve: ulnar nerve (C8, T1)

Opponens pollicis

Action: rotates thumb into opposition with fingers

Origin: flexor retinaculum, tubercles of scaphoid and trapezium, abductor pollicis longus tendon

Insertion: radial side of base of proximal phalanx of thumb

Nerve: median nerve (C8, T1)

Palmar interossei

Action: adducts thumb, index, ring and little fingers
Origin: shaft of metacarpal of digit on which it acts
Insertion: dorsal digital expansion and base of proximal
    phalanx of same digit
Nerve: ulnar nerve (C8, T1)

Palmaris longus

Action: flexes wrist
Origin: medial epicondyle via common flexor tendon
Insertion: flexor retinaculum, palmar aponeurosis
Nerve: median (C7, C8)

Pectineus

Action: flexes and adducts hip
Origin: pecten pubis, iliopectineal eminence, pubic tubercle
Insertion: along a line from lesser trochanter to linea aspera
Nerve: femoral nerve (L2, L3), occasionally accessory
    obturator (L3)

Pectoralis major

Action: adducts, medially rotates, flexes and extends
    shoulder
Origin: clavicular attachment – sternal half of anterior
    surface of clavicle; sternocostal attachment – anterior
    surface of manubrium, body of sternum, upper six costal
    cartilages, sixth rib, aponeurosis of external oblique
    muscle
Insertion: lateral lip of intertubercular sulcus of humerus
Nerve: medial and lateral pectoral nerves (C5–T1)

Pectoralis minor

Action: protracts and medially rotates scapula
Origin: outer surface of third to fifth ribs and adjoining
    intercostal fascia
Insertion: upper surface and medial border of coracoid
    process
Nerve: medial and lateral pectoral nerves (C5–T1)

Peroneus brevis

Action: everts and plantarflexes ankle
Origin: lower two-thirds of lateral surface of fibula,
    intermuscular septa
Insertion: lateral side of base of fifth metatarsal
Nerve: superficial peroneal nerve (L5, S1)

Peroneus longus

Action: everts and plantarflexes ankle
Origin: lateral tibial condyle, upper two-thirds of lateral
    surface of fibula, intermuscular septa
Insertion: lateral side of base of first metatarsal, medial
    cuneiform
Nerve: superficial peroneal nerve (L5, S1)

Peroneus tertius

Action: everts and dorsiflexes ankle
Origin: distal third of medial surface of fibula, interosseous
    membrane, intermuscular septum
Insertion: medial aspect of base of fifth metatarsal
Nerve: deep peroneal nerve (L5, S1)

Piriformis

Action: laterally rotates and abducts hip
Origin: front of second to fourth sacral segments, gluteal
    surface of ilium, pelvic surface of sacrotuberous
    ligament
Insertion: medial side of greater trochanter
Nerve: anterior rami of sacral plexus (L5–S2)

Plantar interossei

Action: adduct third to fifth toes, flex metatarsophalangeal
    joints of lateral three toes
Origin: base and medial side of lateral three toes
Insertion: medial side of base of proximal phalanx of same
    toes and dorsal digital expansions
Nerve: lateral plantar nerve (S2, S3)

Plantaris

Action: plantarflexes ankle, flexes knee
Origin: lateral supracondylar ridge, oblique popliteal ligament
Insertion: tendo calcaneus
Nerve: tibial nerve (S1, S2)

Popliteus

Action: medially rotates tibia, flexes knee
Origin: outer surface of lateral femoral condyle
Insertion: posterior surface of tibia above soleal line
Nerve: tibial nerve (L4–S1)

Pronator quadratus

Action: pronates forearm
Origin: lower quarter of anterior surface of ulna
Insertion: lower quarter of anterior surface of radius
Nerve: anterior interosseous branch of median nerve
    (C7, C8)

Pronator teres

Action: pronates forearm, flexes elbow
Origin: humeral head – medial epicondyle via common flexor
    tendon, intermuscular septum, antebrachial fascia; ulnar
    head – medial part of coronoid process
Insertion: middle of lateral surface of radius
Nerve: median nerve (C6, C7)

Psoas major

Action: flexes hip and lumbar spine
Origin: bodies of T12 and all lumbar vertebrae, bases of
    transverse processes of all lumbar vertebrae, lumbar
    intervertebral discs
Insertion: lesser trochanter
Nerve: anterior rami of lumbar plexus (L1–L3)

Psoas minor (not always present)

Action: flexes trunk (weak)
Origin: bodies of T12 and L1 vertebrae and intervertebral
    discs

Insertion: pecten pubis, iliopubic eminence, iliac fascia
Nerve: anterior primary ramus (L1)

Quadratus femoris

Action: laterally rotates hip
Origin: ischial tuberosity
Insertion: quadrate tubercle midway down intertrochanteric crest
Nerve: nerve to quadratus femoris (L5, S1)

Quadratus lumborum

Action: laterally flexes trunk, extends lumbar vertebrae,
 steadies twelfth rib during deep inspiration
Origin: iliolumbar ligament, posterior part of iliac crest
Insertion: lower border of twelfth rib, transverse processes of
 L1–L4
Nerve: ventral rami of T12 and L1–L3/4

Rectus abdominis

Action: flexes trunk
Origin: symphysis pubis, pubic crest
Insertion: fifth to seventh costal cartilages, xiphoid process
Nerve: ventral rami of T6/7–T12

Rectus capitis anterior

Action: flexes neck
Origin: anterior surface of lateral mass of atlas and root of its
 transverse process
Insertion: occipital bone
Nerve: anterior primary rami (C1, C2)

Rectus capitis lateralis

Action: laterally flexes neck
Origin: transverse process of atlas
Insertion: jugular process of occipital bone
Nerve: ventral rami (C1, C2)

Rectus capitis posterior major

Action: extends and rotates neck
Origin: spinous process of axis

Insertion: lateral part of inferior nuchal line of occipital bone
Nerve: dorsal ramus (C1)

Rectus capitis posterior minor

Action: extends neck
Origin: posterior tubercle of atlas
Insertion: medial part of inferior nuchal line of occipital bone
Nerve: dorsal ramus (C1)

Rectus femoris

Action: extends knee, flexes hip
Origin: straight head – anterior inferior iliac spine; reflected
    head – area above acetabulum, capsule of hip joint
Insertion: base of patella, then forms part of patellar ligament
Nerve: femoral nerve (L2–L4)

Rhomboid major

Action: retracts and medially rotates scapula
Origin: spines and supraspinous ligaments of T2–T5
Insertion: medial border of scapula between root of spine and
    inferior angle
Nerve: dorsal scapular nerve (C4, C5)

Rhomboid minor

Action: retracts and medially rotates scapula
Origin: spines and supraspinous ligaments of C7–T1, lower
    part of ligamentum nuchae
Insertion: medial end of spine of scapula
Nerve: dorsal scapular nerve (C4, C5)

Rotatores

Action: extends vertebral column and rotates thoracic region
Origin: transverse process of each vertebra
Insertion: lamina of vertebra above
Nerve: dorsal rami of spinal nerves

Sartorius

Action: flexes hip and knee, laterally rotates and abducts hip,
    medially rotates tibia on femur

Origin: anterior superior iliac spine and area just below
Insertion: upper part of medial side of tibia
Nerve: femoral nerve (L2, L3)

Scalenus anterior

Action: flexes, laterally flexes and rotates neck, raises first rib during respiration
Origin: anterior tubercles of transverse processes of C3–C6
Insertion: scalene tubercle on inner border of first rib
Nerve: ventral rami (C4–C6)

Scalenus medius

Action: laterally flexes neck, raises first rib during respiration
Origin: transverse processes of atlas and axis, posterior tubercles of transverse processes of C3–C7
Insertion: upper surface of first rib
Nerve: ventral rami (C3–C8)

Scalenus posterior

Action: laterally flexes neck, raises second rib during respiration
Origin: posterior tubercles of transverse processes of C4–C6
Insertion: outer surface of second rib
Nerve: ventral rami (C6–C8)

Semimembranosus

Action: flexes knee, extends hip and medially rotates tibia on femur
Origin: ischial tuberosity
Insertion: posterior aspect of medial tibial condyle
Nerve: tibial division of sciatic nerve (L5–S2)

Semispinalis capitis

Action: extends and rotates head
Origin: transverse processes of C7–T6/7, articular processes of C4–C6
Insertion: between superior and inferior nuchal lines of occipital bone
Nerve: dorsal rami of spinal nerves

Semispinalis cervicis

Action: extends and rotates vertebral column
Origin: transverse processes of T1–T5/6
Insertion: spinous processes of C2–C5
Nerve: dorsal rami of spinal nerves

Semispinalis thoracis

Action: extends and rotates vertebral column
Origin: transverse processes of T6–T10
Insertion: spinous processes of C6–T4
Nerve: dorsal rami of spinal nerves

Semitendinosus

Action: flexes knee, extends hip and medially rotates tibia on femur
Origin: ischial tuberosity
Insertion: upper part of medial surface of tibia
Nerve: tibial division of sciatic nerve (L5–S2)

Serratus anterior

Action: protracts and laterally rotates scapula
Origin: outer surfaces and superior borders of upper eight, nine or ten ribs and intervening intercostal fascia
Insertion: costal surface of medial border of scapula
Nerve: long thoracic nerve (C5–C7)

Soleus

Action: plantarflexes ankle
Origin: soleal line and middle third of medial border of tibia, posterior surface of head and upper quarter of fibula, fibrous arch between tibia and fibula
Insertion: posterior surface of calcaneus
Nerve: tibial nerve (S1, S2)

Spinalis (capitis*, cervicis*, thoracis)

Action: extends vertebral column
Origin: spinalis thoracis – spinous processes of T11–L2
Insertion: spinalis thoracis – spinous processes of upper four to eight thoracic vertebrae

*Spinalis capitis and spinalis cervicis are poorly developed and
  blend with adjacent muscles
Nerve: dorsal rami

Splenius capitis

Action: extends, laterally flexes and rotates neck
Origin: lower half of ligamentum nuchae, spinous processes
  of C7–T3/4 and their supraspinous ligaments
Insertion: mastoid process of temporal bone, lateral third of
  superior nuchal line of occipital bone
Nerve: dorsal rami (C3–C5)

Splenius cervicis

Action: laterally flexes, rotates and extends neck
Origin: spinous processes of T3–T6
Insertion: posterior tubercles of transverse processes of C1–
  C3/4
Nerve: dorsal rami (C5–C7)

Sternocleidomastoid

Action: laterally flexes and rotates neck; anterior fibres flex
  neck, posterior fibres extend neck
Origin: sternal head – anterior surface of manubrium sterni;
  clavicular head – upper surface of medial third of clavicle
Insertion: mastoid process of temporal bone, lateral half of
  superior nuchal line of occipital bone
Nerve: accessory nerve (XI)

Subscapularis

Action: medially rotates shoulder
Origin: medial two-thirds of subscapular fossa and tendinous
  intramuscular septa
Insertion: lesser tubercle of humerus, anterior capsule of
  shoulder joint
Nerve: upper and lower subscapular nerves (C5, C6)

Superior oblique

Action: extends neck
Origin: upper surface of transverse process of atlas

Insertion: superior and inferior nuchal lines of occipital bone
Nerve: dorsal ramus (C1)

Supinator

Action: supinates forearm
Origin: inferior aspect of lateral epicondyle, radial collateral ligament, annular ligament, supinator crest and fossa of ulna
Insertion: posterior, lateral and anterior aspects of upper third of radius
Nerve: posterior interosseous nerve (C6, C7)

Supraspinatus

Action: abducts shoulder
Origin: medial two-thirds of supraspinous fossa and supraspinous fascia
Insertion: capsule of shoulder joint, greater tubercle of humerus
Nerve: suprascapular nerve (C5, C6)

Tensor fascia lata

Action: extends knee, abducts and medially rotates hip
Origin: outer lip of iliac crest between iliac tubercle and anterior superior iliac spine
Insertion: iliotibial tract
Nerve: superior gluteal nerve (L4–S1)

Teres major

Action: extends, adducts and medially rotates shoulder
Origin: dorsal surface of inferior scapular angle
Insertion: medial lip of intertubercular sulcus of humerus
Nerve: lower subscapular nerve (C5–C7)

Teres minor

Action: laterally rotates shoulder
Origin: upper two-thirds of dorsal surface of scapula
Insertion: lower facet on greater tuberosity of humerus, lower posterior surface of capsule of shoulder joint
Nerve: axillary nerve (C5, C6)

Tibialis anterior

Action: dorsiflexes and inverts ankle

Origin: lateral tibial condyle and upper two-thirds of lateral surface of tibia, interosseous membrane

Insertion: medial and inferior surface of medial cuneiform, base of first metatarsal

Nerve: deep peroneal nerve (L4, L5)

Tibialis posterior

Action: plantarflexes and inverts ankle

Origin: lateral aspect of posterior surface of tibia below soleal line, interosseous membrane, upper half of posterior surface of fibula, deep transverse fascia

Insertion: tuberosity of navicular, medial cuneiform, sustentaculum tali, intermediate cuneiform, base of second to fourth metatarsals

Nerve: tibial nerve (L4, L5)

Transversus abdominis

Action: compresses abdominal contents, raises intraabdominal pressure

Origin: lateral third of inguinal ligament, anterior two-thirds of inner lip of iliac crest, thoracolumbar fascia between iliac crest and twelfth rib, lower six costal cartilages where it interdigitates with diaphragm

Insertion: abdominal aponeurosis to linea alba

Nerve: ventral rami of lower six thoracic and first lumbar spinal nerve

Trapezius

Action: upper fibres elevate scapula, middle fibres retract scapula, lower fibres depress scapula, upper and lower fibres together laterally rotate scapula. Also extends and laterally flexes head and neck

Origin: medial third of superior nuchal line, external occipital protuberance, ligamentum nuchae, spinous processes and supraspinous ligaments of C7–T12

Insertion: upper fibres – posterior border of lateral third of clavicle; middle fibres – medial border of acromion, superior lip of crest of spine of scapula; lower fibres – tubercle at medial end of spine of scapula

Nerve: accessory nerve (XI), ventral rami (C3, C4)

Triceps brachii

Action: extends elbow and shoulder

Origin: long head – infraglenoid tubercle of scapula, shoulder capsule; lateral head – above and lateral to spiral groove on posterior surface of humerus; medial head – below and medial to spiral groove on posterior surface of humerus

Insertion: upper surface of olecranon, deep fascia of forearm

Nerve: radial nerve (C6–C8)

Vastus intermedius

Action: extends knee

Origin: upper two-thirds of anterior and lateral surfaces of femur, lower part of lateral intermuscular septum

Insertion: deep surface of quadriceps tendon, lateral border of patella, lateral tibial condyle

Nerve: femoral nerve (L2–L4)

Vastus lateralis

Action: extends knee

Origin: intertrochanteric line, greater trochanter, gluteal tuberosity, lateral lip of linea aspera

Insertion: tendon of rectus femoris, lateral border of patella

Nerve: femoral nerve (L2–L4)

Vastus medialis

Action: extends knee

Origin: intertrochanteric line, spiral line, medial lip of linea aspera, medial supracondylar line, medial intermuscular septum, tendons of adductor longus and adductor magnus

Insertion: tendon of rectus femoris, medial border of patella, medial tibial condyle

Nerve: femoral nerve (L2–L4)

References and Further Reading

Drake, R. L., Vogl, W., & Mitchell, A. W. M. (2014). *Gray's anatomy for students*. Philadelphia: Churchill Livingstone.

O'Brien, M. D. (2010). *Guarantors of 'Brain' 2009–2010. Aids to the examination of the peripheral nervous system* (5th ed.). Edinburgh: W B Saunders.

Palastanga, N., & Soames, R. (2012). *Anatomy and human movement: structure and function* (6th ed.). Edinburgh: Churchill Livingstone.

Standring, S. (2015). *Gray's anatomy: the anatomical basis of clinical practice* (41st ed.). Elsevier.

Thompson, J. C. (2016). *Netter's concise orthopaedic anatomy* (2nd ed.). Philadelphia: Saunders.

Neuromusculoskeletal assessment

Peripheral nerve sensory innervation

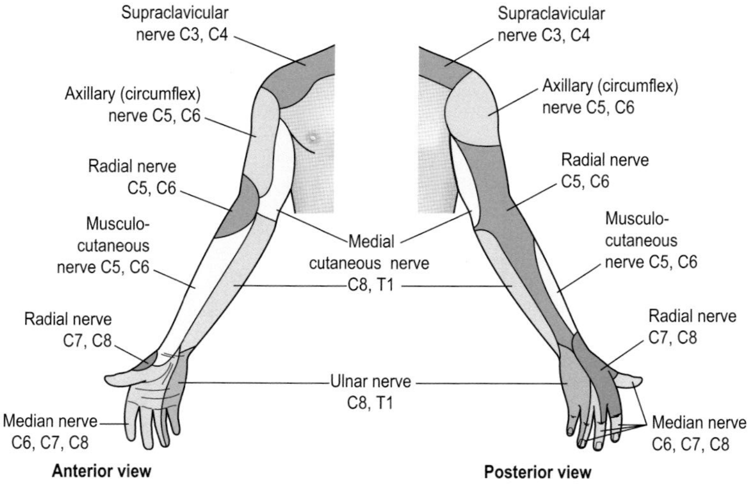

Supraclavicular nerve C3, C4

Axillary (circumflex) nerve C5, C6

Radial nerve C5, C6

Musculo-cutaneous nerve C5, C6

Medial cutaneous nerve C8, T1

Radial nerve C7, C8

Median nerve C6, C7, C8

Ulnar nerve C8, T1

Anterior view

Supraclavicular nerve C3, C4

Axillary (circumflex) nerve C5, C6

Radial nerve C5, C6

Musculo-cutaneous nerve C5, C6

Radial nerve C7, C8

Median nerve C6, C7, C8

Posterior view

Figure 2.1 Cutaneous distribution of the upper limb.

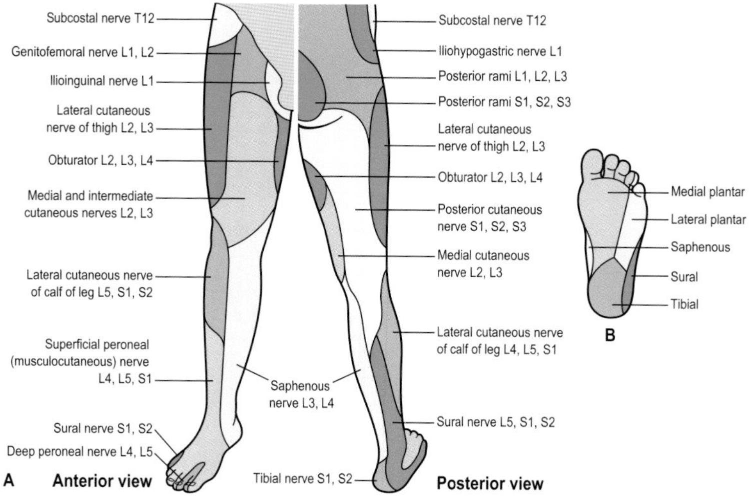

B

Medial plantar
Lateral plantar
Saphenous
Sural
Tibial

Subcostal nerve T12
Iliohypogastric nerve L1
Posterior rami L1, L2, L3
Posterior rami S1, S2, S3
Lateral cutaneous
nerve of thigh L2, L3
Obturator L2, L3, L4
Posterior cutaneous
nerve S1, S2, S3
Medial cutaneous
nerve L2, L3
Lateral cutaneous nerve
of calf of leg L4, L5, S1
Sural nerve L5, S1, S2

Saphenous
nerve L3, L4

Tibial nerve S1, S2

Posterior view

Subcostal nerve T12
Genitofemoral nerve L1, L2
Ilioinguinal nerve L1
Lateral cutaneous
nerve of thigh L2, L3
Obturator L2, L3, L4
Medial and intermediate
cutaneous nerves L2, L3
Lateral cutaneous nerve
of calf of leg L5, S1, S2
Superficial peroneal
(musculocutaneous) nerve
L4, L5, S1
Sural nerve S1, S2
Deep peroneal nerve L4, L5

Saphenous
nerve L3, L4

Tibial nerve S1, S2

A   Anterior view

Figure 2.2 Cutaneous distribution of (**A**) the lower limb and (**B**) the foot.

Dermatomes (from O'Brien 2010, with permission)

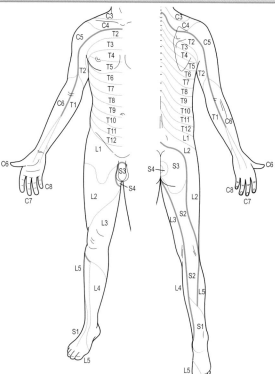

Figure 2.3 Dermatomes of the whole body. The above illustration is used extensively in clinical practice to define the body's dermatomal patterns. It represents the dermatomes as lying between clearly defined boundaries with no overlap between areas. However, it is worth noting that studies have shown that there is significant variability in the pattern of segmental innervation and that the above dermatomes do not always describe the patterns found in a large number of patients. (From O'Brien 2010, Aids to the Examination of the Peripheral Nervous System, 5e, with permission.)

Myotomes

Root	Joint action	Root	Joint action
C1–C2	Cervical flexion	T1	Finger abduction/adduction
C3	Cervical lateral flexion	T2–L1	No muscle test
C4	Shoulder girdle elevation	L2	Hip flexion
C5	Shoulder abduction	L3	Knee extension
C6	Elbow flexion	L4	Ankle dorsiflexion
C7	Elbow extension	L5	Great toe extension
C8	Thumb extension	S1	Ankle eversion/hip extension/ankle plantarflexion/knee flexion
		S2	Knee flexion

Reflexes

Deep tendon reflex	Root	Nerve
Biceps jerk	C5–C6	Musculocutaneous
Brachioradialis jerk	C5–C6	Radial
Triceps jerk	C7–C8	Radial
Knee jerk	L3–L4	Femoral
Ankle jerk	S1–S2	Tibial

When testing reflexes, the patient must be relaxed and the muscle placed on a slight stretch. Look for symmetry of response between reflexes on both sides, and ensure that both limbs are positioned identically. When a reflex is difficult to elicit, a reinforcement manoeuvre can be used to facilitate a stronger response. This is performed while the reflex is being tested. Usually upper-limb reinforcement manoeuvres are used for lower-limb reflexes and vice versa. Examples of reinforcement manoeuvres include clenching the teeth or fists, hooking the hands together by the flexed fingers and pulling one hand against the other (Jendrassik's manoeuvre), crossing the legs at the ankle and pulling one ankle against the other.

Reflexes may be recorded as follows, noting any asymmetry (Petty and Dionne, 2018):

– or 0: absent
– or 1: diminished
+ or 2: average
+ + or 3: exaggerated
+ + + or 4: clonus

An abnormal reflex response may or may not be indicative of a neurological lesion. Findings need to concur with other neurological observations in order to be considered as significant evidence of an abnormality.

An exaggerated response (excessively brisk or prolonged) may simply be caused by anxiety. However, it may also indicate an upper motor neurone lesion, i.e. central damage. Clonus is associated with exaggerated reflexes and also indicates an upper motor neurone lesion. A diminished or absent response may indicate a lower motor neurone lesion, i.e. loss of ankle jerk with lumbosacral disc prolapse.

Other reflexes	Method	Normal response	Abnormal response (indicating possible upper motor neurone lesion)
Plantar (superficial reflex)	Run a blunt object over lateral border of sole of foot from the heel up towards the little toe and across the foot pad	Flexion of toes	Extension of big toe and fanning of other toes (Babinski response)

Continued

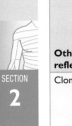

Other reflexes	Method	Normal response	Abnormal response (indicating possible upper motor neurone lesion)
Clonus (tone)	Apply sudden and sustained dorsiflexion to the ankle	Oscillatory beats may occur, but they are not rhythmic or sustained	More than three rhythmic contractions of the plantarflexors
Hoffman reflex	Flick distal phalanx of third or fourth finger downwards	No movement of thumb	Reflex flexion of distal phalanx of thumb

Key features of upper and lower motor neurone lesions

	Upper motor neurone	Lower motor neurone
Muscle tone	Increased	Decreased
Clonus	Present	Absent
Muscle fasciculation	Absent	Present
Tendon reflexes	Increased	Depressed or absent
Plantar response	Extensor (Babinski's sign)	Flexor (normal)
Distribution	Extensor weakness in upper limb and flexor weakness in lower limb Whole limb(s) involved	Weakness of muscle groups innervated by affected spinal segment/root, plexus or peripheral nerve

Upper motor neurone

Origin: cerebral cortex
Terminates: cranial nerve nuclei or spinal cord anterior horn

Lower motor neurone

Origin: cranial nerve motor nuclei or spinal cord anterior horn
Terminates: skeletal muscle motor unit

The Medical Research Council scale for muscle power

Grade	Response
0	No contraction
1	Flicker or trace of contraction
2	Active movement with gravity eliminated
3	Active movement against gravity
4	Active movement against gravity and resistance
5	Normal strength

In addition, Grade 4 movements may be subdivided into:

4−: movement against slight resistance
4: movement against moderate resistance
4+: movement against strong resistance

Medical Research Council 1976 Aids to the investigation of peripheral nerve injuries. London: HMSO. Reproduced with kind permission of the Medical Research Council.

Common locations for palpation of pulses

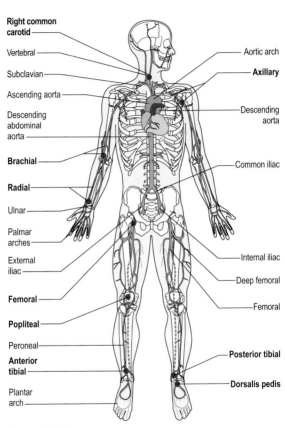

Right common carotid

Vertebral

Subclavian

Ascending aorta

Descending abdominal aorta

Brachial

Radial

Ulnar

Palmar arches

External iliac

Femoral

Popliteal

Peroneal

Anterior tibial

Plantar arch

Aortic arch

Axillary

Descending aorta

Common iliac

Internal iliac

Deep femoral

Femoral

Posterior tibial

Dorsalis pedis

Figure 2.4 Pulse points.

Common carotid	Between the trachea and the sternocleidomastoid muscle
Axillary	Lateral wall of axilla in the groove behind coracobrachialis
Brachial	(a) Between the humerus and biceps on the medial aspect of arm (b) Cubital fossa
Radial	Lateral to flexor carpi radialis tendon
Femoral	In femoral triangle (sartorius, adductor longus and inguinal ligament)
Popliteal	In popliteal fossa. Palpated more easily in prone position with the knee flexed about 45°
Anterior tibial	Above level of ankle joint, between tibialis anterior and extensor hallucis longus tendons
Posterior tibial	Posterior aspect of medial malleolus
Dorsalis pedis	Dorsum of foot, between first and second metatarsal bones

Common musculoskeletal tests

The following section does not contain an exhaustive list of musculoskeletal tests. The tests have been selected according to the frequency of their use in clinical practice and their usefulness in identifying the presence or absence of pathology according to the evidence base. No test is 100% accurate, and interpretation of test findings needs to consider the overall clinical picture.

A brief description of each test is given below. For a fuller description of how each test is performed, please refer to a musculoskeletal assessment textbook.

Shoulder

Active compression test (O'Brien)

Tests: labral pathology, acromioclavicular joint pathology.
Procedure: patient upright with elbow in extension and shoulder in 90° flexion, 10–15° adduction and medial rotation. Stand behind patient, and apply downward force to arm. Repeat with arm in lateral rotation.

Positive sign: pain/increased pain with medial rotation and decreased pain with lateral rotation. Pain inside the glenohumeral joint indicates labral abnormality. Pain over the acromioclavicular joint indicates acromioclavicular joint abnormality.

Anterior drawer test

Tests: anterior shoulder stability.

Procedure: patient supine. Place shoulder in 80–120° abduction, 0–20° forward flexion and 0–30° lateral rotation. Stabilize scapula. Draw humerus anteriorly.

Positive sign: click and/or apprehension.

Anterior slide test

Tests: labral pathology.

Procedure: patient upright with hands on hips, thumbs facing posteriorly. Stand behind patient, and stabilize scapula and clavicle with one hand. With the other hand, apply an anterosuperior force to the elbow while instructing the patient to gently push back against the force.

Positive sign: pain/reproduction of symptoms/click.

Apprehension and relocation test (Fowler's sign)

Tests: glenohumeral joint stability.

Step 1 (Apprehension): patient supine. Abduct shoulder to 90°. Move it into maximum lateral rotation. If movement well tolerated, apply a posteroanterior force to humeral head.

Positive sign: apprehension and pain.

Step 2 (Relocation): At the point where the patient feels pain or apprehension, apply an anteroposterior force to humeral head.

Positive sign: Decrease in pain or apprehension and increased lateral rotation.

Biceps load test I

Tests: superior labral pathology.

Procedure: patient supine with shoulder in 90° abduction, elbow in 90° flexion and forearm supinated. Laterally rotate shoulder until patient becomes apprehensive. Maintain this position. Resist elbow flexion.

Positive sign: pain/apprehension remains unchanged or increases during resisted elbow flexion.

Biceps load test II

Tests: superior labral pathology.

Procedure: patient supine with shoulder in 120° abduction and maximum lateral rotation, elbow in 90° flexion and forearm supinated. Resist elbow flexion.

Positive sign: increased pain during resisted elbow flexion.

Clunk test

Tests: tear of glenoid labrum.

Procedure: patient supine. Abduct shoulder over patient's head. Apply anterior force to posterior aspect of humeral head while rotating humerus laterally.

Positive sign: a clunk or grinding sound and/or apprehension if anterior instability present.

Crank test

Tests: labral pathology.

Procedure: patient sitting or supine with shoulder in 160° flexion in scapular plane. Hold elbow, and apply a longitudinal compressive force to humerus while rotating it medially and laterally.

Positive sign: pain/reproduction of symptoms, with or without click, usually during lateral rotation.

Crossed-arm adduction test (Apley scarf test)

Tests: acromioclavicular joint pathology.

Procedure: patient upright. Horizontally adduct the arm as far as possible.

Positive sign: pain around acromioclavicular joint.

Drop arm test (Codman's test)

Tests: integrity of rotator cuff, particularly supraspinatus.

Procedure: patient standing. Abduct shoulder to 90°. Patient slowly lowers arm to the side.

Positive sign: Inability to lower the arm slowly (i.e. it drops) or severe pain during the movement. Indicates complete/partial rotator cuff tear.

External rotation lag sign

Tests: infraspinatus and supraspinatus integrity.

Procedure: patient upright with shoulder passively elevated to 20° abduction (in the scapular plane) with elbow in 90° flexion. Passively move shoulder into full lateral rotation. Support elbow, and ask patient to hold position.

Positive sign: arm drops into medial rotation.

Hawkins-Kennedy impingement test

Tests: impingement of supraspinatus tendon.

Procedure: patient sitting or standing. Forward flex shoulder to 90° and flex elbow to 90°. Apply passive medial rotation.

Positive sign: reproduction of symptoms.

Hornblower's sign

Tests: teres minor integrity.

Procedure: Patient sitting or standing with arms by side. Patient lifts hands up to mouth.

Positive sign: inability to lift the hand to the mouth without abducting arm first (this compensatory manoeuvre on the affected side is the hornblower's sign).

Jerk test

Tests: posterior shoulder stability.

Procedure: patient sitting. Place shoulder in 90° forward flexion and medial rotation. Apply longitudinal cephalad force to humerus, and move arm into horizontal adduction.

Positive sign: sudden jerk or clunk.

Lift-off test

Tests: subscapularis integrity.

Procedure: patient upright with arm medially rotated behind back. Patient lifts hand away from back.

Positive sign: inability to lift arm indicates tendon rupture.

Load and shift test

Tests: anterior and posterior shoulder stability

Procedure: patient sitting. Stabilize scapula by fixing coracoid process and spine of scapula. Grasp humeral head, and apply a medial, compressive force to seat it in the glenoid fossa (load). Glide the humeral head anteriorly and posteriorly (shift).

Positive sign: increased anterior or posterior glide indicates anterior or posterior instability.

Neer impingement test

Tests: impingement of supraspinatus tendon and/or biceps tendon.

Procedure: patient sitting or standing. Passively elevate arm through forward flexion and medial rotation.

Positive sign: reproduction of symptoms.

Patte's test

Tests: infraspinatus and teres minor integrity.

Procedure: patient sitting. Place shoulder in 90° flexion in the scapular plane and elbow in 90° flexion. Patient rotates arm laterally against resistance.

Positive sign: resistance with pain indicates tendinopathy. Inability to resist with gradual lowering of the arm or forearm indicates tendon rupture.

Posterior drawer test

Tests: posterior shoulder stability.

Procedure: patient supine. Place shoulder in 100–120° abduction and 20–30° forward flexion with elbow flexed to 120°. Stabilize scapula. Medially rotate and forward flex shoulder between 60° and 80° while pushing head of humerus posteriorly.

Positive sign: significant posterior displacement and/or patient apprehension.

Speed's test

Tests: biceps tendon pathology.

Procedure: patient sitting or standing. Forward flex shoulder, supinate forearm and extend elbow. Resist patient's attempt to flex shoulder.

Positive sign: increased pain in bicipital groove.

Sulcus sign

Tests: inferior shoulder stability.

Procedure: patient standing or sitting, arm by side. Grip arm below elbow, and pull distally.

Positive sign: reproduction of symptoms and/or appearance of sulcus under acromion.

Supraspinatus (empty can) test

Tests: supraspinatus tendon pathology; suprascapular nerve neuropathy.

Procedure: patient sitting or standing. Abduct shoulder to 90°. Horizontally flex to 30°, and medially rotate so thumbs point downwards. Resist patient's attempt to abduct.

Positive sign: reproduction of symptoms or weakness.

Yergason's test

Tests: biceps tendon pathology; subacromial impingement.

Procedure: patient sitting or standing with elbow in 90° flexion and forearm pronated. Resist patient's attempts to supinate.

Positive sign: increased pain in bicipital groove.

Elbow

Elbow flexion test

Tests: cubital tunnel (ulnar nerve) syndrome.

Procedure: patient standing or sitting. Fully flex elbows with wrist extended. Hold for 5 minutes.

Positive sign: tingling or paraesthesia in ulnar nerve distribution.

Tennis elbow test (resisted)

Tests: tendinopathy of the wrist extensors involving the common extensor origin at the lateral epicondyle.

Procedure: patient sitting or standing with elbow in full
extension and wrist in full flexion and pronation. Resist
patient's attempts to extend wrist while supporting the
arm under the elbow.

Positive sign: reproduction of symptoms.

Tennis elbow test (passive)

Tests: tendinopathy of the wrist extensors involving the
common extensor origin at the lateral epicondyle.

Procedure: passively extend elbow, pronate forearm and flex
wrist and fingers while palpating lateral epicondyle.

Positive sign: reproduction of symptoms.

Tennis elbow test (resisted middle-finger extension)

Tests: tendinopathy of the wrist extensors involving the
common extensor origin at the lateral epicondyle.

Procedure: resist extension of middle finger distal to PIP
(proximal interphalangeal) joint.

Positive sign: reproduction of symptoms.

Golfer's elbow test (resisted)

Tests: tendinopathy of the wrist flexors involving the common
flexor origin at the medial epicondyle.

Procedure: patient sitting or standing with elbow in full
extension and wrist in full extension and pronation. Resist
patient's attempts to flex wrist while supporting the arm
under the elbow.

Positive sign: reproduction of symptoms.

Golfer's elbow test (passive)

Tests: tendinopathy of the wrist flexors involving the common
flexor origin at the medial epicondyle.

Procedure: passively extend elbow, supinate forearm and extend
wrist and fingers while palpating medial epicondyle.

Positive sign: reproduction of symptoms.

Pinch grip test

Tests: anterior interosseous (median) nerve entrapment.

Procedure: patient pinches tips of index finger and thumb
together.
Positive sign: inability to pinch tip to tip.

Posterolateral pivot shift test

Tests: posterolateral rotatory instability of the elbow and the
integrity of the lateral collateral ligament.
Procedure: patient supine with affected arm overhead and
elbow in 20° flexion and supinated. Stabilize forearm
distal to elbow. Apply a longitudinal compressive force to
the radius and ulna then a valgus stress to the forearm,
while maintaining supination.
Positive sign: apprehension and pain.

Tinel's sign (at elbow)

Tests: point of regeneration of sensory fibres of ulnar
nerve.
Procedure: tap ulnar nerve in groove between olecranon and
medial epicondyle.
Positive sign: tingling sensation in ulnar distribution of
forearm and hand. Furthest point at which abnormal
sensation felt indicates point to which the nerve has
regenerated.

Varus stress test

Tests: stability of lateral collateral ligament.
Procedure: patient sitting. Stabilize upper arm with elbow in
20–30° flexion and humerus in full medial rotation. Apply
adduction/varus force to forearm.
Positive sign: excessive laxity or reproduction of symptoms.

Valgus stress test

Tests: stability of medial collateral ligament.
Procedure: patient sitting. Stabilize upper arm with elbow in
20–30° flexion and humerus in full lateral rotation. Apply
abduction/valgus force to forearm.
Positive sign: increased laxity or reproduction of symptoms.

Wrist and hand

Carpal compression test

Tests: aids diagnosis of carpal tunnel syndrome

Procedure: patient sitting with elbow in extension and supination. Place thumb over course of median nerve, just distal to wrist crease and press firmly for up to 2 minutes.

Positive sign: paraesthesia and pain in median nerve distribution.

Finkelstein test

Tests: tenosynovitis of abductor pollicis longus and extensor pollicis brevis tendons (de Quervain's tenosynovitis).

Procedure: patient makes a fist with thumb inside. Passively move wrist into ulnar deviation.

Positive sign: reproduction of symptoms.

Froment's sign

Tests: ulnar nerve paralysis.

Procedure: grip piece of paper between index finger and thumb. Pull paper away.

Positive sign: flexion of IP (interphalangeal) thumb joint as paper pulled away.

Hand elevation test

Tests: aids diagnosis of carpal tunnel syndrome.

Procedure: patient elevates arm as high as possible and holds for up to 1 minute.

Positive sign: reproduction of symptoms (paraesthesia and/or pain)

Ligamentous instability test for the fingers

Tests: stability of collateral ligaments.

Procedure: apply valgus and varus force to PIP (proximal interphalangeal) or DIP (distal interphalangeal) joint.

Positive sign: increased laxity.

Lunotriquetral ballottement (Reagan's) test

Tests: stability of lunotriquetral ligament.

Procedure: stabilize lunate, and apply posterior and anterior glide to triquetrum and pisiform.

Positive sign: reproduction of symptoms, crepitus or laxity.

Phalen's (wrist flexion) test

Tests: median nerve pathology; carpal tunnel syndrome.

Procedure: place dorsal aspect of hands together with wrists flexed. Hold for 1 minute.

Positive sign: tingling in distribution of median nerve.

Reverse Phalen's test

Tests: median nerve pathology.

Procedure: place palms of hands together with wrists extended. Hold for 1 minute.

Positive sign: tingling in distribution of median nerve.

Scaphoid shift (Watson's) test

Tests: stability of scaphoid.

Procedure: hold wrist in full ulnar deviation and slight extension. With other hand, apply pressure to scaphoid tubercle (palmar aspect) and move wrist into radial deviation and slight flexion.

Positive sign: pain and/or subluxation of scaphoid.

Sweater finger sign

Tests: rupture of flexor digitorum profundus tendon.

Procedure: patient makes a fist.

Positive sign: loss of DIP joint flexion of one of the fingers.

Tinel's sign (at the wrist)

Tests: median nerve pathology; carpal tunnel syndrome.

Procedure: tap over carpal tunnel.

Positive sign: tingling or paraesthesia in median distribution in hand. Furthest point at which abnormal sensation felt indicates point to which the nerve has regenerated.

Thumb grind test

Tests: stability and/or degeneration of the first trapeziometacarpal joint.

Procedure: stabilize wrist and apply longitudinal compressive
force to first metacarpal, then medial and lateral rotation.
Positive sign: pain, crepitus.

Triangular fibrocartilage complex (TFCC) load test

Tests: triangular fibrocartilage complex integrity.
Procedure: hold forearm. With other hand hold wrist in ulnar
deviation, then move it through supination and pronation
while applying a compressive force.
Positive sign: pain, clicking, crepitus.

Wrist flexion and compression test

Tests: aids diagnosis of carpal tunnel syndrome.
Procedure: patient sitting with elbow in extension and
supination. Flex wrist to 60°, place thumb over course of
median nerve, just distal to wrist crease and press firmly
for up to 30 seconds.
Positive sign: reproduction of symptoms (paraesthesia and/or
pain).

Pelvis

Compression test

Tests: sprain of posterior sacroiliac joint or ligaments.
Procedure: patient supine or side lying. Push right and left
ASIS (anterior superior iliac spine) towards each other.
Positive sign: reproduction of symptoms.

Gaenslen's test

Tests: sacroiliac joint.
Procedure: patient supine with leg hanging over side of plinth.
Patient hugs contralateral knee to chest. Place one hand
above knee of extended leg and other hand over knee of
flexed leg. Apply an opposing force to each leg
simultaneously.
Positive sign: reproduction of pain.

Gapping test (distraction)

Tests: sprain of anterior sacroiliac joint or ligaments.

Procedure: patient supine. Push right and left ASIS apart.
Positive sign: reproduction of symptoms.

Gillet's test

Tests: sacroiliac joint dysfunction.
Procedure: patient standing. Palpate PSIS (posterior superior iliac spine) and sacrum at same level. Patient flexes hip and knee on side being palpated while standing on opposite leg. Repeat test on other side and compare.
Positive sign: if the PSIS on the side tested does not move downwards in relation to the sacrum, it indicates hypomobility on that side.

Piedallu's sign (sitting flexion)

Tests: movement of sacrum on ilia.
Procedure: patient sitting. Left and right PSIS are palpated while patient forward flexes.
Positive sign: one side moves higher than the other, indicating hypomobility on that side.

Shear test

Tests: sacroiliac joint
Procedure: patient prone. Apply downward and superior pressure to sacral base.
Positive sign: reproduction of pain.

Standing flexion

Tests: movement of ilia on sacrum.
Procedure: patient standing. Left and right PSIS are palpated while patient forward flexes.
Positive sign: one side moves higher than the other, indicating hypomobility on that side.

Supine to sit (long sitting) test

Tests: sacroiliac joint dysfunction caused by pelvic torsion or rotation.

Procedure: patient supine. Note level of inferior borders of medial malleoli. Patient sits up and relative position of malleoli noted.

Positive sign: one leg moves up more than the other.

Thigh thrust test (femoral shear test)

Tests: sacroiliac joint.

Procedure: patient supine. Place hip and knee in 90° flexion. Place one hand on top of flexed knee and the other under the sacrum. Apply longitudinal force down femur.

Positive sign: reproduction of pain.

Hip

FABER test (Patrick's test)

Tests: hip joint or sacroiliac joint dysfunction; spasm of iliopsoas muscle.

Procedure: patient supine. Place foot of test leg on opposite knee. Gently lower knee of test leg.

Positive sign: knee remains above the opposite leg; pain or spasm.

Leg length test

Tests: leg-length discrepancy.

Procedure: patient supine. Measure between the anterior superior iliac spine and the medial or lateral malleolus.

Positive sign: a difference of more than 1.3 cm is considered significant.

Ober's sign

Tests: tensor fascia lata and iliotibial band contractures.

Procedure: patient side lying with hip and knee of lower leg flexed. Stabilize pelvis. Passively abduct and extend upper leg with knee extended or flexed to 90°, then allow it to drop towards plinth.

Positive sign: upper leg remains abducted and does not lower to plinth.

Quadrant test

Tests: intra-articular hip joint pathology.

Procedure: patient supine. Place hip in full flexion and adduction. Abduct hip in a circular arc, maintaining full flexion, while applying a longitudinal compressive force.

Positive sign: pain, locking, crepitus, clicking, apprehension.

Thomas test

Tests: hip flexion contracture.

Procedure: patient supine. Patient hugs one knee to chest.

Positive sign: opposite leg lifts off plinth.

Modified Thomas test

Tests: flexibility of iliopsoas, rectus femoris and tensor fascia lata/iliotibial band.

Procedure: patient lies supine towards the bottom edge of the plinth allowing lower leg to hang off the end. Patient hugs knees to chest, then lowers contralateral leg as far as possible.

Positive sign: leg unable to reach neutral position (contact with plinth): tightness of iliopsoas or rectus femoris. To differentiate, passively flex knee: increased hip flexion indicates rectus femoris; unchanged hip flexion indicates iliopsoas. Increased hip abduction indicates tightness of tensor fascia lata/iliotibial band.

Trendelenburg's sign

Tests: stability of the hip, strength of hip abductors (gluteus medius).

Procedure: patient stands on one leg.

Positive sign: pelvis on opposite side drops.

Weber-Barstow Manoeuvre

Tests: leg length asymmetry.

Procedure: patient supine with hips and knees flexed. Hold patient's feet palpating medial malleoli with thumbs. Patient lifts pelvis off bed and returns to starting position.

Passively extend legs, and compare relative position of medial malleoli.

Positive sign: leg length asymmetry.

Knee

Abduction (valgus) stress test

Tests: full knee extension: anterior cruciate ligament, medial quadriceps expansion, semimembranosus muscle, medial collateral ligaments, posterior oblique ligament, posterior cruciate ligament, posteromedial capsule.

20–30° flexion: medial collateral ligament, posterior oblique ligament, posterior cruciate ligament, posteromedial capsule.

Procedure: patient supine. Stabilize ankle, and apply medial pressure (valgus stress) to knee joint at 0° and then at 20–30° extension.

Positive sign: excessive movement compared with opposite knee.

Adduction (varus) stress test

Tests: full knee extension: cruciate ligaments, lateral gastrocnemius muscle, lateral collateral ligament, arcuate-popliteus complex, posterolateral capsule, iliotibial band, biceps femoris tendon.

20–30° flexion: lateral collateral ligament, arcuate-popliteus complex, posterolateral capsule, iliotibial band, biceps femoris tendon.

Procedure: patient supine. Stabilize ankle. Apply lateral pressure (varus stress) to knee joint at 0° and then at 20–30° extension.

Positive sign: excessive movement compared with opposite knee.

Anterior drawer test

Tests: anterior cruciate ligament, posterior oblique ligament, arcuate-popliteus complex, posteromedial and posterolateral capsules, medial collateral ligament, iliotibial band.

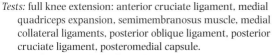

Procedure: patient supine with hips flexed to 45° and knee flexed to 90°. Stabilize foot. Apply posteroanterior force to tibia.

Positive sign: tibia moves more than 6 mm on the femur.

Apley's test

Tests: distraction for ligamentous injury; compression for meniscus injury.

Procedure: patient prone with knee flexed to 90°. Medially and laterally rotate tibia – first with distraction and then compression.

Positive sign: pain.

Brush test

Tests: mild effusion.

Procedure: patient supine with knee extended as much as possible. Stroke medial side of patella from just below joint line up to suprapatellar pouch two or three times. Use opposite hand to stroke down lateral side of patella.

Positive sign: fluid travels to medial side and appears as bulge below distal border of patella.

External rotation recurvatum test

Tests: posterolateral rotary stability in knee extension.

Procedure: patient supine. Hold heel, and place knee in 30° flexion. Slowly extend knee while palpating posterolateral aspect of knee.

Positive sign: excessive hyperextension and lateral rotation palpated.

Hughston plica test

Tests: inflammation of suprapatellar plica.

Procedure: patient supine. Flex and medially rotate knee while applying medial glide to patella and palpating medial femoral condyle. Passively extend and flex knee.

Positive sign: popping of plica band over femoral condyle, tenderness.

Lachman's test

Tests: anterior cruciate ligament, posterior oblique ligament, arcuate-popliteus complex.

Procedure: patient supine with knee flexed 0–30°. Stabilize femur. Apply posteroanterior force to tibia.

Positive sign: soft end feel or excessive movement.

McConnell test for chondromalacia patellae

Tests: chondromalacia patellae.

Procedure: patient high sitting with femur laterally rotated. Isometric quad contractions are performed at 0°, 30°, 60°, 90° and 120° of knee flexion for 10 seconds. If pain is produced with any of these movements, repeat test with patella pushed medially.

Positive sign: decrease in symptoms with medial glide.

McMurray test

Tests: medial meniscus and lateral meniscus injury.

Procedure: patient supine with test knee completely flexed. To test the medial meniscus, laterally rotate knee and passively extend to 90° while palpating joint line. To test the lateral meniscus, repeat test with the knee in medial rotation.

Positive sign: a snap or click.

Patella apprehension (Fairbank's) test

Tests: patellar subluxation or dislocation.

Procedure: patient supine with knee in 30° flexion and quads relaxed. Passively glide patella laterally.

Positive sign: patient apprehension or excessive movement.

Patellofemoral grind test (Clarke's sign)

Tests: whether the patellofemoral joint is the origin of pain.

Procedure: patient supine or long sitting with knees extended. Place web space of thumb over superior border of patella. Apply downward and inferior pressure to the patella as the patient contracts quadriceps muscles.

Positive sign: reproduction of symptoms.

Pivot shift test

Tests: integrity of anterior cruciate ligament.

Procedure: patient supine. Place the hip in 45° flexion and
30° abduction, and flex the knee to 45°. One hand
supports the knee while applying a valgus force to the
proximal fibula. The other hand cradles the foot while
applying an internal rotation force to the tibia, using the
foot as a lever. As both forces are applied, slowly extend
the knee.

Positive sign: A 'jerk' or 'clunk' as the tibia reduces backwards
at approximately 30° flexion.

*Note: this test is easier to perform and more accurate under
general anaesthetic.*

Posterior drawer test

Tests: posterior cruciate ligament, arcuate-popliteus complex,
posterior oblique ligament, anterior cruciate ligament.

Procedure: patient supine with hips flexed to 45° and knee
flexed to 90°. Stabilize foot. Apply anteroposterior force to
tibia.

Positive sign: excessive movement.

Posterior sag sign

Tests: posterior cruciate ligament, arcuate-popliteus complex,
posterior oblique ligament, anterior cruciate ligament.

Procedure: patient supine with hips flexed to 45° and knee
flexed to 90° with feet on plinth.

Positive sign: tibia drops posteriorly.

Slocum test for anterolateral rotary instability

Tests: anterior and posterior cruciate ligaments, posterolateral
capsule, arcuate-popliteus complex, lateral collateral
ligaments, iliotibial band.

Procedure: patient supine with hips flexed to 45° and knee
flexed to 90°. Place foot in 30° medial rotation and
stabilize. Apply posteroanterior force to tibia.

Positive sign: excessive movement on lateral side when
compared with opposite knee.

Slocum test for anteromedial rotary instability

Tests: medial collateral ligament, posterior oblique ligament, posteromedial capsule, anterior cruciate ligament.

Procedure: patient supine with hips flexed to 45° and knee flexed to 90°. Place foot in 15° lateral rotation and stabilize. Apply posteroanterior force to tibia.

Positive sign: excessive movement on medial side when compared with opposite knee.

Weight-bearing/rotation meniscal test (Thessaly or Disco test)

Tests: integrity of the menisci.

Procedure: patient standing on affected leg in slight knee flexion (20°). Hold patient's hands for support. Patient rotates body from left to right several times.

Positive sign: pain, catching, locking or apprehension.

Ankle and foot

Anterior drawer sign

Tests: medial and lateral ligament integrity.

Procedure: patient prone with knee flexed. Apply posteroanterior force to talus with ankle in dorsiflexion and then plantarflexion.

Positive sign: excessive anterior movement (both ligaments affected) or movement on one side only (ligament on that side affected).

Syndesmosis squeeze test

Tests: integrity of interosseous membrane/ligaments.

Procedure: patient long sitting or supine. Squeeze the fibula and tibia together above the midpoint of the calf.

Positive sign: reproduction of pain.

Talar tilt

Tests: adduction: mainly integrity of calcaneofibular ligament but also anterior talofibular ligament. *Abduction:* integrity of deltoid ligament.

Procedure: patient prone, supine or side lying with knee flexed. Tilt talus into abduction and adduction with patient's foot in neutral.

Positive sign: excessive movement.

Thompson's test

Tests: Achilles tendon rupture.

Procedure: patient prone with feet over edge of plinth. Squeeze calf muscles.

Positive sign: absence of plantarflexion.

Common vascular tests

Adson's manoeuvre

Tests: thoracic outlet syndrome.

Procedure: patient sitting. Patient turns head toward test arm and extends head. Laterally rotate and extend shoulder and arm while palpating radial pulse. Patient takes a deep breath and holds it.

Positive sign: disappearance of radial pulse.

Elevated arm stress test (Ross test)

Tests: thoracic outlet syndrome.

Procedure: patient stands and abducts arm to 90°, laterally rotates shoulders and flexes elbow to 90°. Patient opens and closes hands for 3 minutes.

Positive sign: inability to keep arms in starting position, pain, heaviness or weakness in arm, tingling in hand.

Homan's test

Tests: deep vein thrombophlebitis.

Procedure: patient supine. Passive dorsiflexion of ankle with knee extended.

Positive sign: pain in the calf.

Provocation elevation test

Tests: thoracic outlet syndrome.

Procedure: patient standing with arms above head. Patient opens and closes hands 15 times.
Positive sign: fatigue, cramping, tingling.

Neurological tests

Finger–nose test

Hold your finger about an arm's length from the patient. Ask the patient to touch your finger with the index finger and then touch the nose, repeating the movement back and forth. Patients may demonstrate past pointing (missing your finger) or intention tremor.

Indicates: possible cerebellar dysfunction.

Heel–shin test

With the patient lying down, ask the patient to place one heel on the opposite knee and then run the heel down the tibial shaft toward the ankle and back again. Patients may demonstrate intention tremor, an inability to keep the heel on the shin or uncoordinated movements.

Indicates: possible cerebellar dysfunction.

Hoffman reflex

Flick the distal phalanx of the patient's third or fourth finger. Look for any reflex flexion of the patient's thumb.

Indicates: possible upper motor neurone lesion.

Joint position sense

Test the most distal joint of the limb, i.e. distal phalanx of the index finger or interphalangeal joint of the hallux. With the patient's eyes open, demonstrate the movement. To test, ask the patient to close the eyes. Hold the joint to be tested at the sides between two fingers, and move it up and down. Ask the patient to identify the direction of movement, ensuring that you are not moving more proximal joints or brushing against the neighbouring toes or fingers. If there is impairment, test more proximal joints.

Indicates: loss of proprioception.

Light touch

Use a wisp of cotton wool. With the patient's eyes open, demonstrate what you are going to do. To test, ask the patient to close the eyes. Stroke the patient's skin with the cotton wool at random points, asking the patient to indicate every time he or she feels the touch.

Indicates: altered touch sensation.

Pin prick

Use a disposable neurological pin which has a sharp end and a blunt end. With the patient's eyes open, demonstrate what you are going to do. To test, ask the patient to close the eyes. Test various areas of the limb randomly using sharp and blunt stimuli, and ask the patient to tell you which sensation he or she feels.

Indicates: altered pain sensation.

Plantar reflex (Babinski)

Apply a firm pressure along the lateral aspect of the sole of the foot and across the base of the toes, observing the big toe. If the big toe flexes, the response is normal. If the big toe extends and the other toes spread, it indicates a positive Babinski's sign.

Indicates: A positive Babinski's sign signifies a possible upper motor neurone lesion.

Rapidly alternating movement

Ask the patient to hold out one hand palm up and then alternately slap it with the palmar and then dorsal aspect of the fingers of the other hand. Where there is a loss of rhythm and fluency, it is referred to as dysdiadochokinesia. For the lower limbs, ask the patient to tap first one foot on the floor and then the other.

Indicates: possible cerebellar dysfunction.

Romberg's test

Patient stands with feet together and eyes open. Ask the patient to close the eyes (ensuring that you can support the patient if he or she falls). Note any excessive postural sway or loss of balance.

Indicates: proprioceptive or vestibular deficit if the patient falls only when he or she closes the eyes.

Temperature

A quick test involves using a cold object such as a tuning fork and asking the patient to describe the sensation when applied to various parts of the body. For more formal testing, two test tubes are filled with cold and warm water, and patients are asked to distinguish between the two sensations.

Indicates: altered temperature sensation.

Two-point discrimination

Requires a two-point discriminator, a device similar to a pair of blunted compasses. With the patient's eyes open, demonstrate what you are going to do. Ask the patient to close the eyes. Alternately touch the patient with either one prong or two. Reduce the distance between the prongs until the patient can no longer discriminate between being touched by one prong or two prongs. Varies according to skin thickness, but normal young patients can distinguish a separation of approximately 5 mm in the index finger and approximately 4 cm in the legs. Compare left with right.

Indicates: impaired sensory function.

Vibration sense

Use a 128-Hz tuning fork. Ask the patient to close the eyes. Place the tuning fork on a bony prominence or on the fingertips or toes. The patient should report feeling the vibration and not simply the contact of the tuning fork. If in doubt, apply the tuning fork and then stop it vibrating suddenly by pinching it between your fingers, and see if the patient can correctly identify when it stops vibrating.

Indicates: altered vibration sense.

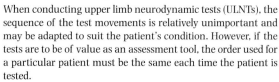
Neurodynamic tests

Upper limb neurodynamic tests

When conducting upper limb neurodynamic tests (ULNTs), the sequence of the test movements is relatively unimportant and may be adapted to suit the patient's condition. However, if the tests are to be of value as an assessment tool, the order used for a particular patient must be the same each time the patient is tested.

For all the upper limb neurodynamic tests, you may wish to place the patient's head in contralateral cervical flexion before you do the test and then instruct the patient to bring his or her head back to midline at the end of the sequence.

ULNT 1: Median nerve bias

ULNT 1 (Fig. 2.5) consists of:

* Neutral position of patient on couch in supine
* Fixing shoulder to prevent shoulder elevation during abduction [1]
* Shoulder joint abduction [2]
* Wrist and finger extension [3]
* Forearm supination [3]
* Shoulder lateral rotation [4]
* Elbow extension [5]

Sensitizing test: cervical lateral flexion away from the symptomatic side [6].

Desensitizing test: cervical lateral flexion toward the symptomatic side.

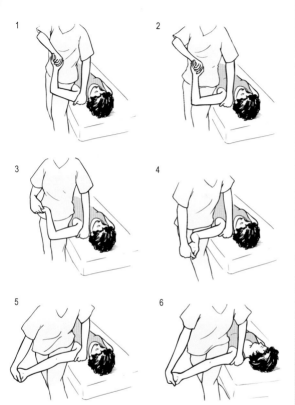

Figure 2.5 (1–6) Upper limb neurodynamic test 1.

ULNT 2a: Median nerve bias

ULNT 2a (Fig. 2.6) consists of:

- Neutral position of patient on couch in supine
- Shoulder girdle depression [1, 2]
- Elbow extension [3]
- Lateral rotation of whole arm [4]

125

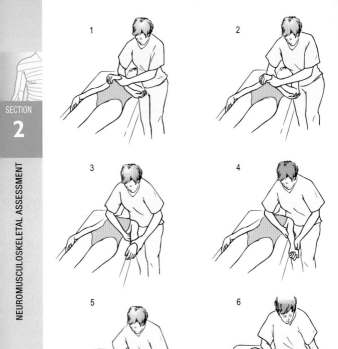

Figure 2.6 (1–6) Upper limb neurodynamic test 2a.

- Wrist, finger and thumb extension [5]
- Abduction of shoulder [6]

Sensitizing test: cervical lateral flexion away from the symptomatic side.

Desensitizing tests: cervical lateral flexion toward the
symptomatic side or release of the shoulder girdle
depression.

ULNT 2b: Radial nerve bias

ULNT 2b (Fig. 2.7) consists of:

* Neutral position of patient on couch in supine
* Shoulder girdle depression [1]
* Elbow extension [2]
* Medial rotation of whole arm [3]
* Wrist, finger and thumb flexion [4]
* Shoulder abduction

Sensitizing test: cervical lateral flexion away from the
symptomatic side.

Desensitizing tests: cervical lateral flexion toward the
symptomatic side or release of the shoulder girdle
depression.

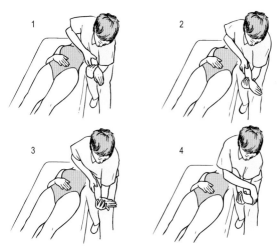

Figure 2.7 (1–4) Upper limb neurodynamic test 2b.

ULNT 3: Ulnar nerve bias

ULNT 3 (Fig. 2.8) consists of:

- Neutral position of patient on couch in supine
- Shoulder girdle stabilised [1]
- Wrist and finger extension [1]
- Forearm pronation [2]
- Elbow flexion [3]
- Shoulder lateral rotation [4]
- Shoulder abduction [5]

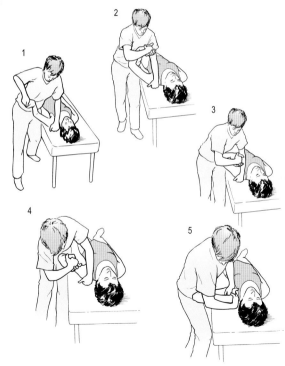

Figure 2.8 (1–5) Upper limb neurodynamic test 3.

Sensitizing test: cervical lateral flexion away from the symptomatic side.

Desensitizing tests: cervical lateral flexion toward the symptomatic side or release of the shoulder girdle depression.

Slump test (Fig. 2.9)

Starting position: patient sits upright with knee crease at the edge of plinth and hands behind back [1]. The slump test consists of:

- Spinal slump [2]
- Cervical flexion [3]
- Knee extension [4]
- Release neck flexion [5]

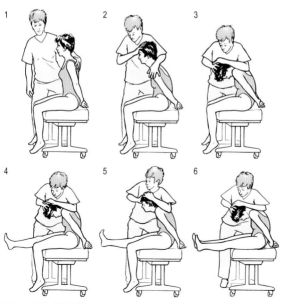

Figure 2.9 (1–6) Slump test.

The steps can be performed in any order.

Additional movements: add dorsiflexion or plantarflexion with knee extension; bilateral knee extension [6], hip abduction (obturator nerve bias), hip medial rotation, hip flexion.

Positive test: development of pain or discomfort in mid-thoracic area, behind the knees or in the hamstrings; restriction of knee extension while slumped with the neck flexed; restriction of dorsiflexion while slumped with the neck flexed. Release of neck flexion decreases pain or increases range of knee extension and/or dorsiflexion.

Desensitizing test: a decrease in pain or increase in range of knee extension and/or dorsiflexion with cervical extension.

Straight leg raise (Fig. 2.10)

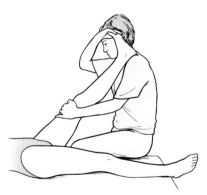

Figure 2.10 Straight leg raise.

Starting position: patient lies supine. The test consists of passive hip flexion with the knee in extension.

Normal response: feeling of stretch or tingling in posterior leg. Altered responses can be determined by comparing one side with the other.

Sensitizing tests: dorsiflexion, hip adduction, hip medial rotation, neck flexion and trunk lateral flexion.

Additional sensitizing tests: Add ankle dorsiflexion and forefoot eversion (tibial nerve bias), ankle plantarflexion and forefoot inversion (common peroneal nerve bias), dorsiflexion and inversion (sural nerve bias).

Passive neck flexion (Fig. 2.11)

Starting position: patient lies supine. The test consists of passive neck flexion.

Normal response: full, pain-free movement.

Sensitizing tests: straight leg raise, upper limb neurodynamic tests.

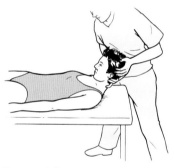

Figure 2.11 **Passive neck flexion.**

Femoral Nerve Slump Test (Fig. 2.12)

Starting position: patient in side lying with symptomatic side uppermost. Holds bottom knee to chest and flexes neck.

Sensitizing tests: the uppermost knee is passively flexed and the hip extended.

Positive test: reproduction of symptoms in anterior thigh.

Desensitizing test: cervical extension reduces symptoms.

Additional sensitizing tests: hip medial or lateral rotation and/ or hip abduction/adduction.

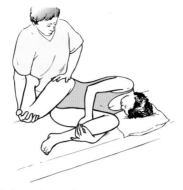

Figure 2.12 Femoral nerve slump test.

Cranial nerves

The cranial nerves form part of the peripheral nervous system and originate from the brain. Each nerve is named according to its function or appearance and is numbered using Roman numerals I to XII. The numbers roughly correspond to their position as they descend from just above the brainstem (I and II), through the midbrain (III and IV), pons (V to VII) and medulla (VIII to XII).

Name	Function	Test	Abnormal signs
Olfactory (I)	Smell	Identify a familiar odour, e.g. coffee, orange, tobacco, with one nostril at a time	Partial or total loss of smell Altered or increased sense of smell
Optic (II)	Sight	Visual acuity: read with one eye covered Peripheral vision: detect objects or movement from the corner of the eye with the other eye covered	Visual field defects, loss of visual acuity, colour-blindness
Oculomotor (III)	Movement of eyelid and eyeball, constriction of pupil, lens accommodation	Follow the examiner's finger, which moves up and down and side to side, keeping the head in mid-position	Squint, ptosis, diplopia, pupil dilation
Trochlear (IV)	Movement of eyeball upwards	As for oculomotor	Diplopia, squint
Trigeminal (V)	Mastication, sensation for eye, face, sinuses and teeth	Test facial sensation Clench teeth (the examiner palpates the masseter and temporalis muscles)	Trigeminal neuralgia, loss of mastication and sensation in eye, face, sinuses and teeth

Continued

133

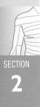

Name	Function	Test	Abnormal signs
Abducens (VI)	Movement of eyeball into abduction, controls gaze	As for oculomotor	Gaze palsy
Facial (VII)	Facial movements, sensation and taste for anterior two-thirds of tongue, secretion of saliva and tears	Test ability to move the face, e.g. close eyes tightly, wrinkle brow, whistle, smile, show teeth	Bell's palsy, loss of taste and ability to close eyes
Vestibulocochlear (VIII)	Hearing, balance	Examiner rubs index finger and thumb together noisily beside one ear and silently beside the other. Patient identifies the noisy side	Tinnitus, deafness, vertigo, ataxia, nystagmus
Glossopharyngeal (IX)	Sensation and taste for posterior third of tongue, swallow, salivation, regulation of blood pressure	Swallow Evoke the gag reflex by touching the back of the throat with a tongue depressor	Loss of tongue sensation and taste, reduced salivation, dysphagia

Vagus (X)	Motor and sensation for heart, lungs, digestive tract and diaphragm, secretion of digestive fluids, taste, swallow, hiccups	As for glossopharyngeal	Vocal cord paralysis, dysphagia, loss of sensation from internal organs
Accessory (XI)	Motor to soft palate, larynx, pharynx, trapezius and sternocleidomastoid	Rotate neck to one side and resist flexion, i.e. contract sternocleidomastoid. Shrug shoulders against resistance	Paralysis of innervated muscles
Hypoglossal (XII)	Tongue control and strap muscles of neck	Stick out the tongue. Push tongue into the left and right side of the cheek	Dysphagia, dysarthria, difficulty masticating

Glossary of terms used to evaluate clinical tests

True positive

The patient has the disease, and the test is positive.

False positive

The patient does not have the disease, but the test is positive.

True negative

The patient does not have the disease, and the test is negative.

False negative

The patient has the disease, but the test is negative.

Sensitivity and specificity

The *sensitivity* of a clinical test refers to the ability of the test to correctly identify those patients with the disease (true positive rate). In other words, if the test is highly sensitive, then a negative result will almost certainly mean that the patient does not have the disease.

The *specificity* of a clinical test refers to the ability of the test to correctly identify those patients without the disease (true negative rate). In other words, if a test is highly specific, then a positive result would indicate that the patient is likely to have the disease.

A way of remembering this is by remembering the terms *Snout* and *Spin*:

SnOut – in a sensitive *(Sn)* test, a negative *(n)* result rules *Out* disease.

SpIn – in a specific *(Sp)* test, a positive *(p)* result rules *In* disease.

Positive predictive value (PPV)

The PPV answers the question: "If the test result is positive, what is the probability that the patient actually has the disease?"

For example, if a test has a small positive predictive value (i.e. PPV = 15%), it indicates that many of the positive results from the testing procedure are false positives.

Negative predictive value (NPV)

The NPV answers the question: "If the test result is negative, what is the probability that the patient does not have the disease?"

For example, if a test has a high negative predictive value (i.e. NPV = 95%), we can be confident that the negative results from the testing procedure are true negatives.

Common postures (from Kendall et al. 2005, with permission of Williams & Wilkins)

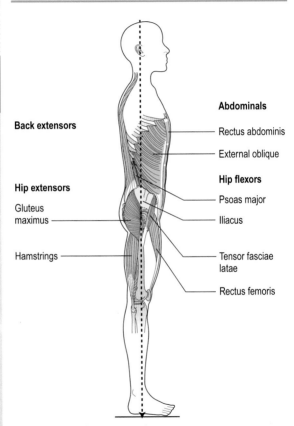

Back extensors

Abdominals

Rectus abdominis

External oblique

Hip flexors

Psoas major

Iliacus

Tensor fasciae latae

Rectus femoris

Hip extensors

Gluteus maximus

Hamstrings

Figure 2.13 Ideal alignment – side view.

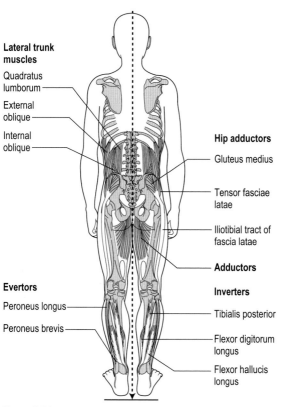

Lateral trunk muscles

Quadratus lumborum

External oblique

Internal oblique

Hip adductors

Gluteus medius

Tensor fasciae latae

Iliotibial tract of fascia latae

Adductors

Evertors

Peroneus longus

Peroneus brevis

Inverters

Tibialis posterior

Flexor digitorum longus

Flexor hallucis longus

Figure 2.14 Ideal alignment – posterior view.

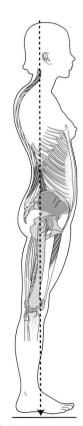

Figure 2.15 Kyphosis-lordosis posture.

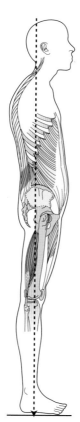

Figure 2.16 Sway-back posture.

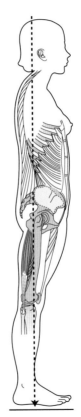

Figure 2.17 Flat-back posture.

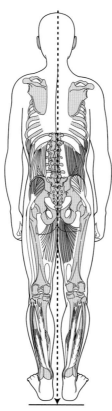

Figure 2.18 Faulty alignment – posterior view.

Ideal alignment

Anteriorly, the abdominal muscles pull upward and the hip flexors pull downward. Posteriorly, the back muscles pull upward and the hip extensors pull downward. Thus, the abdominal and hip extensor muscles work together to tilt the pelvis posteriorly; the back and hip flexor muscles work together to tilt the pelvis anteriorly.

Kyphosis-lordosis posture

Short and strong: neck extensors and hip flexors. The low back is strong and may or may not develop shortness.

Elongated and weak: neck flexors, upper back erector spinae and external oblique. Hamstrings are slightly elongated but may or may not be weak.

Swayback posture

Short and strong: hamstrings and upper fibres of internal oblique. Strong but not short: lumbar erector spinae.

Elongated and weak: one-joint hip flexors, external oblique, upper back extensors and neck flexors.

Flat-back posture

Short and strong: hamstrings and often the abdominals.

Elongated and weak: one-joint hip flexors.

Faulty alignment: posterior view

Short and strong: right lateral trunk muscles, left hip abductors, right hip adductors, left peroneus longus and brevis, right tibialis posterior, right flexor hallucis longus, right flexor digitorum longus. The left tensor fascia lata is usually strong, and there may be tightness in the iliotibial band.

Elongated and weak: left lateral trunk muscles, right hip abductors (especially posterior gluteus medius), left hip adductors, right peroneus longus and brevis, left tibialis posterior, left flexor hallucis longus, left flexor digitorum longus. The right tensor fascia lata may or may not be weak.

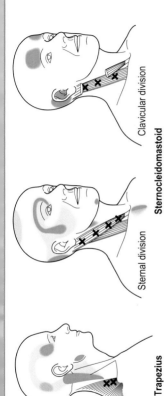

Clavicular division

Sternal division

Sternocleidomastoid

TrP₁

Trapezius

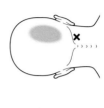

Semispinalis cervicis

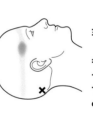

Semispinalis capitis

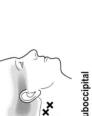

Suboccipital

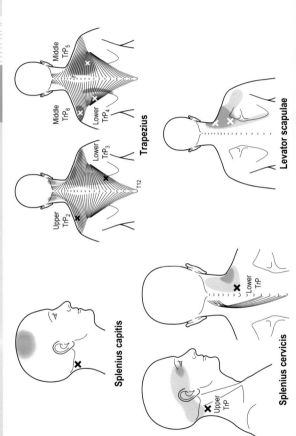

Trapezius

Levator scapulae

Splenius capitis

Splenius cervicis

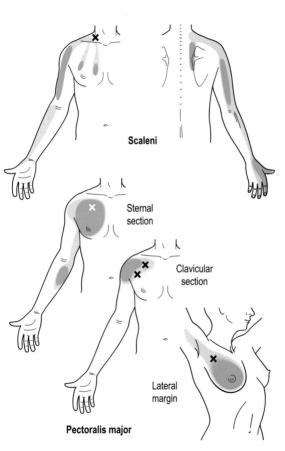

Scaleni

Sternal section

Clavicular section

Lateral margin

Pectoralis major

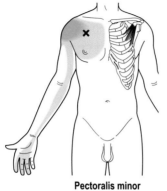

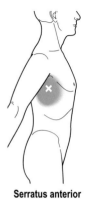

Pectoralis minor

Serratus anterior

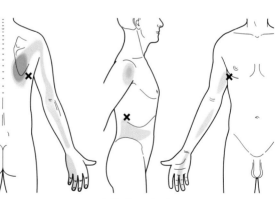

Latissimus dorsi

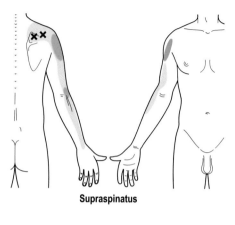

Supraspinatus

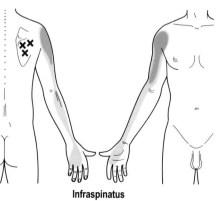

Infraspinatus

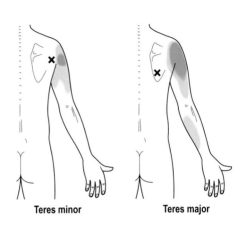

Teres minor

Teres major

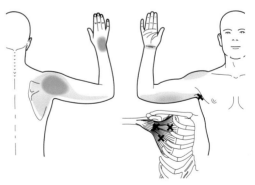

Subscapularis

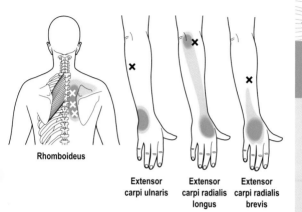

Rhomboideus

Extensor
carpi ulnaris

Extensor
carpi radialis
longus

Extensor
carpi radialis
brevis

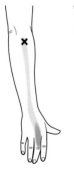

Middle finger

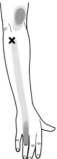

Ring finger

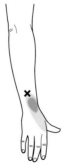

Extensor indicis

Finger extensors

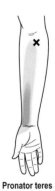

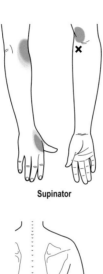

Supinator

Pronator teres

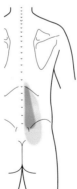

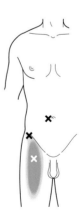

Iliopsoas

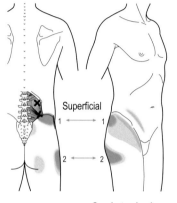

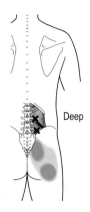

Quadratus lumborum

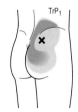

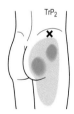

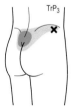

Gluteus medius

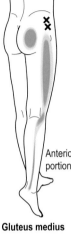

Anterior
portion

Gluteus medius

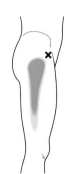

TrP₁

TrP₂

Piriformis

Tensor fasciae latae

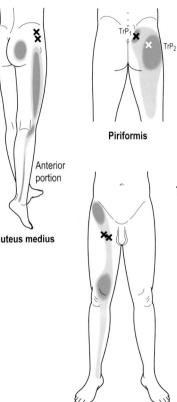

Adductor brevis

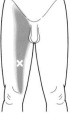

Adductor magnus

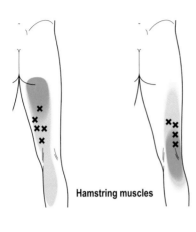

Hamstring muscles

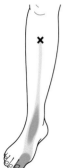

Tibialis anterior

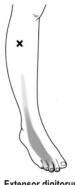

Extensor digitorum longus

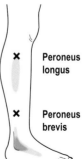

Peroneus longus

Peroneus brevis

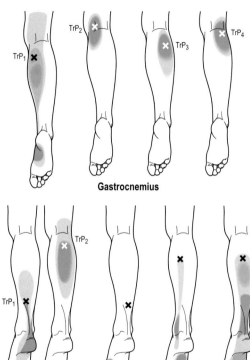

Gastrocnemius

Soleus **Flexor hallucis longus** **Flexor digitorum longus** **Tibialis posterior**

Normal joint range of movement

Shoulder

Flexion	160–180°
Extension	50–60°
Abduction	170–180°
Medial rotation	70–90°
Lateral rotation	80–100°

Elbow

Flexion	140–150°
Extension	0°
Pronation	80–90°
Supination	80–90°

Wrist

Flexion	70–80°
Extension	60–80°
Radial deviation	15–25°
Ulnar deviation	30–40°

Hip

Flexion	120–125°
Extension	15–30°
Abduction	30–50°
Adduction	20–30°
Medial rotation	25–40°
External rotation	40–50°

Knee

Flexion	130–140°
Extension	0°

Ankle

Dorsiflexion	15–20°
Plantarflexion	50–60°
Inversion	30–40°
Eversion	15–20°

Normal ranges of movement vary greatly between individuals. The above figures represent average ranges of movement.

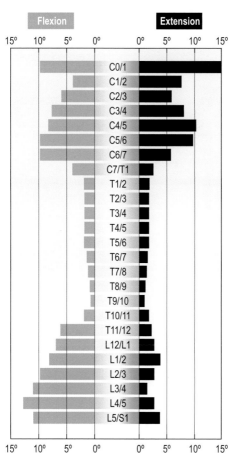

Figure 2.19 Spinal flexion and extension.

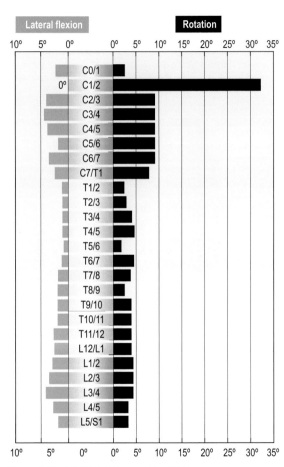

Figure 2.20 Spinal lateral flexion and rotation.

Close packed positions and capsular patterns for selected joints

Joint	Close packed position	Capsular pattern*
Temporomandibular	Clenched teeth	Opening mouth
Cervical spine	Extension (also applies to thoracic and lumbar spine)	Side flexion and rotation equally limited; flexion is full but painful, extension is limited
Glenohumeral	Abduction and lateral rotation	Lateral rotation then abduction then medial rotation
Humeroulnar	Extension	Flexion then extension
Radiocarpal	Extension with radial deviation	Flexion and extension equally limited
Trapeziometacarpal	None	Abduction and extension, full flexion
Metacarpophalangeal interphalangeal	*Metacarpophalangeal* Flexion (fingers) Opposition (thumb) *Interphalangeal* Extension	Flexion then extension
Hip	Extension and medial rotation	Flexion, abduction and medial rotation (order may vary) Extension is slightly limited
Knee	Extension and lateral rotation of tibia	Flexion then extension
Talocrural	Dorsiflexion	Plantarflexion then dorsiflexion
Subtalar	Inversion	Inversion

Joint	Close packed position	Capsular pattern*
Mid-tarsal	Inversion (also applies to tarsometatarsal)	Dorsiflexion, plantarflexion, adduction and medial rotation
First metatarsophalangeal	*Metatarsophalangeal* Extension	Extension then flexion
	Interphalangeal Extension	

*Movements are listed in order of restriction, from the most limited to the least limited.
Data from Cyriax (1982) and Magee (2014).

Classification of ligament and muscle sprains

Ligament sprains

Grade I/mild sprain

Few ligament fibres torn, stability maintained.

Grade II/moderate sprain

Partial rupture, increased laxity but no gross instability.

Grade III/severe sprain

Complete rupture, gross instability.

Muscle strains

Grade I/mild strain

Few muscle fibres torn, minimum loss of strength and pain on muscle contraction.

Grade II/moderate strain

Approximately half of muscle fibres torn, significant muscle weakness and loss of function. Moderate to severe pain on isometric contraction.

Grade III/severe strain

Complete tear of the muscle, significant muscle weakness and severe loss of function. Minimum to no pain on isometric contraction.

Windows of achievement for gross motor developmental milestones

Motor activity	Approximate age
Rolling	2–9 months
Sitting without support	4–9 months
Crawling/creeping	5–14 months
Pulling up to supported stand	8–12 months
Standing with assistance	5–12 months
Cruising (i.e. walking holding onto furniture)	8–12 months
Walking with assistance	6–14 months
Standing alone	7–17 months
Walking alone	8–18 months
Kicking/throwing a ball	2 years
Running	2 years
Jumping with both feet	2–3 years
Mounting/descending stairs alone	3–4 years
Riding a tricycle	3 years
Catching a ball	3–5 years
Balancing on one leg	3–5 years
Hopping	3–4 years
Skipping	4–5 years
Riding a bicycle	4–8 years

Date compiled from Dosman et al, 2012; Gallahue et al, 2012; Haibach et al, 2011; WHO Multicentre Growth Reference Study Group, 2006.

Joint hypermobility assessment

Beighton hypermobility score (Beighton et al 1973)

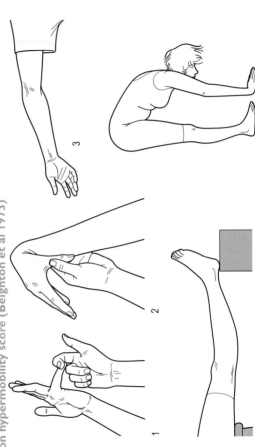

Nine-point Beighton hypermobility score

The ability to:	Right	Left
1 Passively extend the fifth metacarpophalangeal joint to ≥90°	1	1
2 Passively appose the thumb to the anterior aspect of the forearm	1	1
3 Passively hyperextend the elbow to ≥10°	1	1
4 Passively hyperextend the knee to ≥10°	1	1
5 Actively place the hands flat on the floor without bending the knees	1	
TOTAL	9	

One point is given for each side for manoeuvres 1–4 so that the hypermobility score will have a maximum of 9 points if all are positive.

It is generally considered that hypermobility is present if 5 or more of the 9 possible points are scored. In children, a positive score is at least 6 out of 9 points.

It is worth noting that the Beighton scoring system is useful as a quick screening tool. However, it is limited to a small selection of joints. Clinicians are advised to examine other joints (e.g. shoulders, cervical and thoracic spine, toes and feet) for further evidence of hypermobility.

Five-part questionnaire for identifying joint hypermobility (Hakim & Graham 2003)

An answer of 'Yes' to two or more of the questions gives a high prediction of the presence of hypermobility. It does not mean that the person has hypermobility syndrome.

1. Can you now (or could you ever) place your hands flat on the floor without bending your knees?
2. Can you now (or could you ever) bend your thumb to touch your forearm?
3. As a child, did you amuse your friends by contorting your body into strange shapes, OR could you do the splits?

4. As a child or teenager, did your shoulder or kneecap dislocate on more than one occasion?
5. Do you consider yourself double-jointed?

Complex regional pain syndrome

Budapest criteria: clinical diagnostic criteria for complex regional pain syndrome (Harden et al 2007)

To make the clinical diagnosis, the following criteria must be met:

1. Continuing pain, which is disproportionate to any inciting event
2. Must report at least one symptom in three of the four following categories:
   * *Sensory:* Reports of hyperesthesia and/or allodynia
   * *Vasomotor:* Reports of temperature asymmetry and/or skin colour changes and/or skin colour asymmetry
   * *Sudomotor/oedema:* Reports of oedema and/or sweating changes and/or sweating asymmetry
   * *Motor/trophic:* Reports of decreased range of motion and/or motor dysfunction (weakness, tremor, dystonia) and/or trophic changes (hair, nails, skin)
3. Must display at least one sign at time of evaluation in two or more of the following categories:
   * *Sensory:* Evidence of hyperalgesia (to pinprick) and/or allodynia (to light touch and/or temperature sensation and/or deep somatic pressure and/or joint movement)
   * *Vasomotor:* Evidence of temperature asymmetry (>1°C) and/or skin colour changes and/or asymmetry
   * *Sudomotor/oedema:* Evidence of oedema and/or sweating changes and/or sweating asymmetry
   * *Motor/trophic:* Evidence of decreased range of motion and/or motor dysfunction (weakness, tremor, dystonia) and/or trophic changes (hair, nails, skin)
4. There is no other diagnosis that better explains the signs and symptoms.

Distribution of referred pain (Tortora & Derrickson 2017)

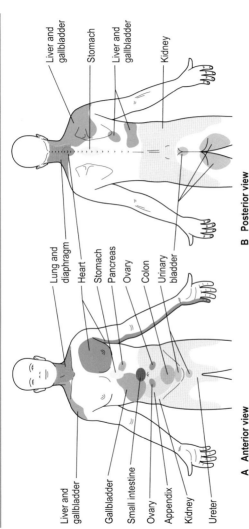

A Anterior view

B Posterior view

Figure 2.22 **A** and **B** Common patterns of referred pain of visceral origin.

Cauda equina syndrome (from National Institute for Health and Care Excellence, Clinical Knowledge Summaries 2017, with permission)

- Severe or progressive bilateral neurological deficit of the legs, such as major motor weakness with knee extension, ankle eversion, or foot dorsiflexion.
- Recent-onset urinary retention (caused by bladder distension because the sensation of fullness is lost) and/or urinary incontinence (caused by loss of sensation when passing urine).
- Recent-onset faecal incontinence (due to loss of sensation of rectal fullness).
- Perianal or perineal sensory loss (saddle anaesthesia or paraesthesia).
- Unexpected laxity of the anal sphincter.

Spinal fracture (from National Institute for Health and Care Excellence, Clinical Knowledge Summaries 2017, with permission)

- Sudden onset of severe central spinal pain that is relieved by lying down
- There may be a history of major trauma (such as a road traffic collision or fall from a height), minor trauma, or even just strenuous lifting in people with osteoporosis or those who use corticosteroids
- Structural deformity of the spine (such as a step from one vertebra to an adjacent vertebra) may be present
- There may be point tenderness over a vertebral body

Cancer (from National Institute for Health and Care Excellence, Clinical Knowledge Summaries 2017, with permission)

- The person being 50 years of age or more
- Gradual onset of symptoms

- Severe unremitting pain that remains when the person is supine, aching night pain that prevents or disturbs sleep, pain aggravated by straining (for example, when defecating, or when coughing or sneezing), and thoracic pain.
- Localized spinal tenderness
- No symptomatic improvement after 4 to 6 weeks of conservative low back pain therapy
- Unexplained weight loss
- Past history of cancer –breast, lung, gastrointestinal, prostate, renal, and thyroid cancers are more likely to metastasize to the spine

Infection (such as discitis, vertebral osteomyelitis, or spinal epidural abscess) (from National Institute for Health and Care Excellence, Clinical Knowledge Summaries 2017, with permission)

- Fever
- Tuberculosis, or recent urinary tract infection
- Diabetes
- History of intravenous drug use
- HIV infection, use of immunosuppressants, or the person is otherwise immunocompromised

Inflammatory disease (axial spondyloarthritis) (from Spondyloarthritis in over 16s: diagnosis and management 2017, with permission)

Inflammatory disease should be suspected if the person's low back pain started before 45 years of age, has lasted for longer than 3 months and four or more of the following additional criteria are also present:

- low back pain that started before 35 years of age (this further increases the likelihood that back pain is due to spondyloarthritis compared with low back pain that started between 35 and 44 years of age)
- waking during the second half of the night because of symptoms
- buttock pain
- improvement with movement

- improvement within 48 hours of taking nonsteroidal anti-inflammatory drugs (NSAIDs)
- a first-degree relative with spondyloarthritis
- current or past arthritis
- current or past enthesitis
- current or past psoriasis

Psychosocial yellow flags (Accident Compensation Corporation 2004, with permission)

Attitudes and beliefs about back pain

- Belief that pain is harmful or disabling resulting in fear-avoidance behaviour, e.g., the development of guarding and fear of movement
- Belief that a pain must be abolished before attempting to return to work or normal activity
- Expectation of increased pain with activity or work, lack of ability to predict capability
- Catastrophizing, thinking the worst, misinterpreting bodily symptoms
- Belief that pain is uncontrollable
- Passive attitude to rehabilitation behaviours
- Use of extended rest, disproportionate 'downtime'
- Reduced activity level with significant withdrawal from activities of daily living
- Irregular participation or poor compliance with physical exercise, tendency for activities to be in a 'boom-bust' cycle
- Avoidance of normal activity and progressive substitution of lifestyle away from productive activity
- Report of extremely high intensity of pain, e.g. above 10, on a 0–10 visual analogue scale
- Excessive reliance on use of aids or appliances
- Sleep quality reduced since onset of back pain
- High intake of alcohol or other substances (possibly as self-medication), with an increase since onset of back pain
- Smoking

Compensation issues

- Lack of financial incentive to return to work
- Delay in accessing income support and treatment cost, disputes over eligibility
- History of claim/s due to other injuries or pain problems
- History of extended time off work due to injury or other pain problem (e.g. more than 12 weeks)
- History of previous back pain, with a previous claim/s and time off work
- Previous experience of ineffective case management (e.g. absence of interest, perception of being treated punitively)

Diagnosis and treatment

- Health professional sanctioning disability, not providing interventions that will improve function
- Experience of conflicting diagnoses or explanations for back pain, resulting in confusion
- Diagnostic language leading to catastrophizing and fear (e.g. fear of ending up in a wheelchair)
- Dramatization of back pain by health professional producing dependency on treatments, and continuation of passive treatment
- Number of times visited health professional in last year (excluding the present episode of back pain)
- Expectation of a 'techno-fix', e.g. requests to treat as if body were a machine
- Lack of satisfaction with previous treatment for back pain
- Advice to withdraw from job

Emotions

- Fear of increased pain with activity or work
- Depression (especially long-term low mood), loss of sense of enjoyment
- More irritable than usual
- Anxiety about and heightened awareness of body sensations (includes sympathetic nervous system arousal)
- Feeling under stress and unable to maintain sense of control

- Presence of social anxiety or disinterest in social activity
- Feeling useless and not needed

Family

- Overprotective partner/spouse, emphasizing fear of harm or encouraging catastrophizing (usually well-intentioned)
- Solicitous behaviour from spouse (e.g. taking over tasks)
- Socially punitive responses from spouse (e.g. ignoring, expressing frustration)
- Extent to which family members support any attempt to return to work
- Lack of support person to talk to about problems

Work

- History of manual work, notably from the following occupational groups:
  - Fishing, forestry and farming workers
  - Construction, including carpenters and builders
  - Nurses
  - Truck drivers
  - Labourers
- Work history, including patterns of frequent job changes, experiencing stress at work, job dissatisfaction, poor relationships with peers or supervisors, lack of vocational direction
- Belief that work is harmful; that it will do damage or be dangerous
- Unsupportive or unhappy current work environment
- Low educational background, low socioeconomic status
- Job involves significant biomechanical demands, such as lifting, manual handling heavy items, extended sitting, extended standing, driving, vibration, maintenance of constrained or sustained postures, inflexible work schedule preventing appropriate breaks
- Job involves shift work or working unsociable hours
- Minimal availability of selected duties and graduated return to work pathways, with unsatisfactory implementation of these

- Negative experience of workplace management of back pain (e.g., absence of a reporting system, discouragement to report, punitive response from supervisors and managers)
- Absence of interest from employer

Remember the key question to bear in mind while conducting these clinical assessments is 'What can be done to help this person experience less distress and disability?'

How to judge if a person is at risk for long-term work loss and disability

A person may be at risk if:

- There is a cluster of a few very salient factors
- There is a group of several less important factors that combine cumulatively

There is good agreement that the following factors are important and consistently predict poor outcomes:

- Presence of a belief that back pain is harmful or potentially severely disabling
- Fear-avoidance behaviour (avoiding a movement or activity due to misplaced anticipation of pain) and reduced activity levels
- Tendency to low mood and withdrawal from social interaction
- An expectation that passive treatments rather than active participation will help

Suggested questions (to be phrased in treatment provider's own words):

- Have you had time off work in the past with back pain?
- What do you understand is the cause of your back pain?
- What are you expecting will help you?
- How is your employer responding to your back pain? Your coworkers? Your family?
- What are you doing to cope with back pain?
- Do you think that you will return to work? When?

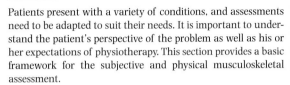

Musculoskeletal assessment

Patients present with a variety of conditions, and assessments need to be adapted to suit their needs. It is important to understand the patient's perspective of the problem as well as his or her expectations of physiotherapy. This section provides a basic framework for the subjective and physical musculoskeletal assessment.

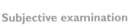

Subjective examination

Body chart

Location of current symptoms
Type of pain
Depth, quality, intensity of symptoms
Intermittent or constant
Abnormal sensation (e.g. pins and needles, numbness)
Relationship of symptoms
Check other relevant regions

Behaviour of symptoms

Aggravating factors
Easing factors
Severity
Irritability
Daily activities/functional limitations
24-hour behaviour (night pain)
Stage of the condition

Special questions

Red flags
Dizziness or other symptoms of vertebrobasilar insufficiency
    (diplopia, drop attacks, dysarthria, dysphagia, nausea)
General health (e.g. smoking, alcohol, physical activity)

History of present condition

Mechanism of injury
History of each symptomatic area

Relationship of onset of each symptomatic area
Change of each symptom since onset
Previous episodes of present complaint
Previous treatment and outcome
Recent X-rays or investigations

Past medical history

Relevant medical history
THREAD (**T**hyroid disorders, **H**eart problems, **R**heumatoid
    arthritis, **E**pilepsy, **A**sthma or other respiratory problems,
    Diabetes)
Osteoporosis
Family history

Drug history

Current medication
Steroids
Anticoagulants

Social history

Age and gender
Home and work situation
Dependents
Hobbies and activities
Exercise

Yellow flags

Physical examination

Observation
Posture
Function
Gait
Structural abnormalities
Muscle bulk and tone
Soft tissues

Active and passive joint movements

Joint integrity tests (i.e. valgus and varus stress test)

Muscle tests

Muscle strength
Muscle control and stability
Muscle length
Isometric muscle testing

Neurological tests

Integrity of the nervous system
• dermatomes
• reflexes
• myotomes
Sensitivity of the nervous system
• straight leg raise
• slump test
• slump knee bend
• passive neck flexion
• upper limb neurodynamic tests
Neurological tests (e.g. coordination, balance)

Other tests (e.g. vascular, cranial)

Palpation

Skin and superficial soft tissue
Muscle and tendon
Nerve
Ligament
Joint
Bone
Pulses

Passive accessory movements

References and Further Reading

Accident Compensation Corporation (2004). *New Zealand acute low back pain guide: Incorporating the guide to assessing psychosocial yellow flags in acute low back pain*. New Zealand: ACC. www.acc.co.nz.

Beighton, P. H., et al. (1973). Articular mobility in an African population. *Annals of the Rheumatic Diseases, 32,* 413–418.

Brukner, P., & Khan, K. (2016). *Clinical sports medicine: Injuries* (5th ed., Vol. 1). Sydney: McGraw-Hill.

Cyriax, J. (1982). *Textbook of orthopaedic medicine* (8th ed., Vol. 1). Diagnosis of soft tissue lesions. London: Baillière Tindall.

Day, R., Fox, J., & Paul-Taylor, G. (2009). *Neuromusculoskeletal clinical tests: A clinician's guide.* Edinburgh: Churchill Livingstone.

Dosman, C. F., Andrews, D., & Goulden, K. J. (2012). Evidence-based milestone ages as a framework for developmental surveillance. *Paediatric Child Health, 17*(10), 561–568.

Gallahue, D. L., Ozmun, J. C., & Goodway, J. D. (2012). *Understanding motor development: infants, children, adolescents, adults* (7th ed.). New York: McGraw-Hill.

Grahame, R., Bird, H. A., Child, A., Dolan, A. L., Edwards-Fowler, A., Ferrell, W., et al. (2000). The British society special interest group on heritable disorders of connective tissue criteria for the benign joint hypermobility syndrome. The revised (Brighton 1998) criteria for the diagnosis of the BJHS. *Journal of Rheumatology, 27*(7), 1777–1779.

Greenhalgh, S., & Selfe, J. (2006). *Red flags: A guide to identifying serious pathology of the spine.* Edinburgh: Churchill Livingstone.

Greenhalgh, S., & Selfe, J. (2010). *Red flags II: A guide to solving serious pathology of the spine.* Edinburgh: Churchill Livingstone.

Grieve, G. P. (1991). *Mobilisation of the spine: A primary handbook of clinical method* (5th ed.). Edinburgh: Churchill Livingstone.

Haibach, P. S., Reid, G., & Collier, D. H. (2011). Motor learning and development. Champaign, IL: Human Kinetics.

Hakim, A. J., & Grahame, R. (2003). A simple questionnaire to detect hypermobility: an adjunct to the assessment of patients with diffuse musculoskeletal pain. *International Journal of Clinical Practice, 57,* 163–166.

Hamblen, D. L., & Simpson, H. W. (2009). *Adams's outline of orthopaedics* (14th ed.). Edinburgh: Churchill Livingstone.

Harden, R. N., Bruehl, S., Stanton-Hicks, M., & Wilson, P. R. (2007). Proposed new diagnostic criteria for complex regional pain syndrome. *Pain Medicine (Malden, Mass.), 8*(4), 326–331.

Hattam, P., & Smeatham, A. (2010). *Special tests in musculoskeletal examination: An evidence-based guide for clinicians.* Edinburgh: Churchill Livingstone.

Hengeveld, E., & Banks, K. (2013). *Maitland's Peripheral Manipulation: Management of neuromusculoskeletal disorders* (5th ed., Vol. 2). Edinburgh: Churchill Livingstone.

Hengeveld, E., Banks, K., & English, K. (2013). *Maitland's Vertebral Manipulation: Management of neuromusculoskeletal disorders* (8th ed., Vol. 1). Edinburgh: Churchill Livingstone.

Innes, J. A., Dover, A. R., & Fairhurst, K. (2018). *Macleod's clinical examination* (14th ed.). Edinburgh: Elsevier.

Kendall, F. P., McCreary, E. K., Provance, P. G., Rodgers, M. M., & Romani, W. A. (2005). *Muscles: Testing and function with posture and pain* (5th ed.). Baltimore: Lippincott Williams & Wilkins.

Kendall, F. P., et al. (2005). *Muscles testing and function in posture and pain* (5th ed.). Baltimore: Williams & Wilkins.

Magee, D. J. (2014). *Orthopedic physical examination* (6th ed.). St Louis: Saunders.

Malanga, G. A., & Mautner, K. (2016). *Musculoskeletal physical examination: An evidence based approach* (2nd ed.). Philadelphia: Elsevier.

Medical Research Council (1976). *Aids to the investigation of peripheral nerve injuries.* London: HMSO.

Middleditch, A., & Oliver, J. (2005). *Functional anatomy of the spine* (2nd ed.). Edinburgh: Butterworth Heinemann.

National Institute for Health and Care Excellence (2017) Spondyloarthritis in over 16s: diagnosis and management. NICE guideline [NG65]. Available at https://www.nice.org.uk/search?q=ng65.

National Institute for Health and Care Excellence, Clinical Knowledge Summaries 2017 *Sciatica (Lumbar Radiculopathy)* Available at https://cks.nice.org.uk/sciatica-lumbar-radiculopathy.

Petty, N. J., & Dionne, R. (2018). *Neuromusculoskeletal examination and assessment: A handbook for therapists* (5th ed.). Elsevier.

Reese, N. B., & Bandy, W. D. (2016). *Joint range of motion and muscle length testing* (3rd ed.). Philadelphia: WB Saunders.

Shacklock, M. (2005). *Clinical neurodynamics: A new system of musculoskeletal treatment.* Edinburgh: Butterworth Heinemann.

Simons, D. G., Travell, J. G., & Simons, L. S. (1998). *Travell and Simon's myofascial pain and dysfunction: The trigger point manual* (2nd ed., Vol. 1). Upper half of body. Baltimore: Lippincott Williams & Wilkins.

Todd, N. V., & Dickson, R. A. (2016). Standards of care in cauda equina syndrome. *British Journal of Neurosurgery, 30*(5), 518–522.

Tortora, G. J., & Derrickson, B. H. (2017). *Principles of anatomy and physiology* (15th ed.). Singapore: John Wiley & Sons.

Travell, J. G., & Simons, D. G. (1991). *Myofascial pain and dysfunction: The trigger point manual* (Vol. 2). The lower extremities. Baltimore: Lippincott Williams & Wilkins.

WHO Multicentre Growth Reference Study Group. (2006). WHO Motor Development Study: Windows of achievement for six gross motor development milestones. *Acta Paediatrica Supplement, 450,* 86–95.

Neurology

SECTION 3

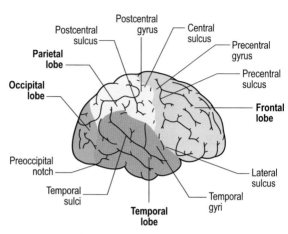

Figure 3.1 Lateral view of right cerebral hemisphere.

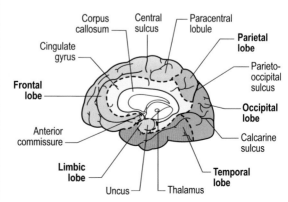

Figure 3.2 Medial view of right cerebral hemisphere.

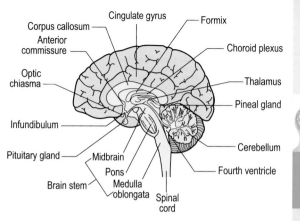

Figure 3.3 Mid-sagittal section of the brain.

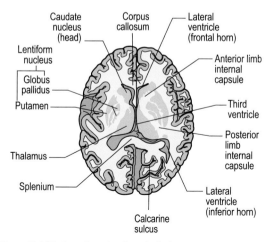

Figure 3.4 Horizontal section through the brain.

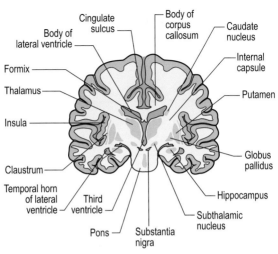

Figure 3.5 Coronal section of the brain.

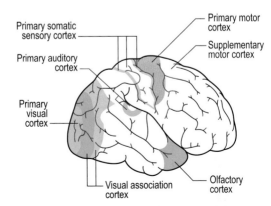

Figure 3.6 Lateral view of sensory and motor cortical areas.

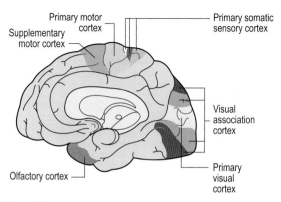

Figure 3.7 Medial view of sensory and motor cortical areas.

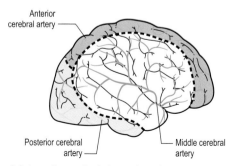

Figure 3.8 Lateral view of right hemisphere showing territories supplied by the cerebral arteries.

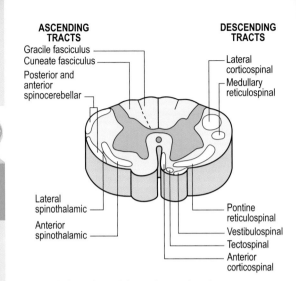

Figure 3.9 Ascending and descending spinal cord tracts.

Ascending tracts	Descending tracts
Gracile fasciculus – proprioception and discriminative touch in legs and lower trunk	Lateral corticospinal – voluntary movements
Cuneate fasciculus – proprioception and discriminative touch in arms and upper trunk	Medullary retrospinal – locomotion and posture
Posterior and anterior spinocerebellar – reflex and proprioception	Pontine reticulospinal – locomotion and posture
Lateral spinothalamic – pain and temperature	Vestibulospinal – balance and antigravity muscles
Anterior spinothalamic – light touch	Tectospinal – orientates head to visual stimulation
	Anterior corticospinal – voluntary movements

Signs and symptoms of cerebrovascular lesions

Middle cerebral artery (MCA)

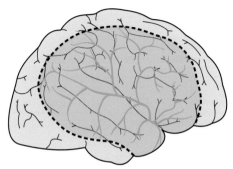

Figure 3.10 Middle cerebral artery The middle cerebral artery arises from the internal carotid artery. The proximal part supplies a large portion of the frontal, parietal and temporal lobes. The deep branches supply the basal ganglia (corpus striatum and globus pallidus), internal capsule and thalamus.

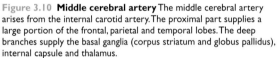

Signs and symptoms	Structures involved
Contralateral weakness/paralysis of face, arm, trunk and leg	Motor cortex (precentral gyrus)
Contralateral sensory impairment/loss of face, arm, trunk and leg	Somatosensory cortex (postcentral gyrus)
Expressive aphasia (Broca's aphasia)	Motor speech area of Broca (dominant frontal lobe)
Receptive aphasia (Wernicke's aphasia)	Sensory speech area of Wernicke (dominant parietal/temporal lobe)
Neglect of contralateral side, dressing and constructional apraxia, geographical agnosia, anosognosia	Parietal lobe (nondominant lobe)

Signs and symptoms	Structures involved
Homonymous hemianopia (often upper homonymous quadrantanopia)	Optic radiation – temporal fibres
Ocular deviation	Frontal lobe
Gait disturbance	Frontal lobe (usually bilateral)
Pure motor hemiplegia	Posterior limb of internal capsule and adjacent corona radiata
Pure sensory syndrome	Ventral posterior nucleus of thalamus

Anterior cerebral artery (ACA)

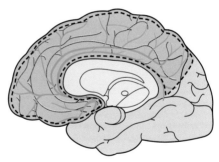

Figure 3.11 **Anterior cerebral artery** The anterior cerebral artery arises from the internal carotid artery and is connected by the anterior communicating artery. It follows the curve of the corpus callosum and supplies the medial aspect of the frontal and parietal lobes, corpus callosum, internal capsule and basal ganglia (caudate nucleus and globus pallidus).

Signs and symptoms	Structures involved
Contralateral hemiplegia/ hemiparesis (lower limb > upper limb)	Motor cortex

Signs and symptoms	Structures involved
Contralateral sensory loss/impairment (lower limb > upper limb)	Somatosensory cortex
Urinary incontinence	Superior frontal gyrus (bilateral)
Contralateral grasp reflex	Frontal lobe
Akinetic mutism, whispering, apathy	Frontal lobe (bilateral)
Ideomotor apraxia, tactile agnosia, agraphia of the left hand	Corpus callosum
Spastic paresis of lower limb	Bilateral motor leg area
Pathological grasp reflex, alien-hand phenomenon	Supplementary motor area, corpus callosum, cingulate gyrus
Gait apraxia	Corpus callosum, cingulate gyrus (usually bilateral)
Impaired memory, confabulation	Basal forebrain

Posterior cerebral artery (PCA)

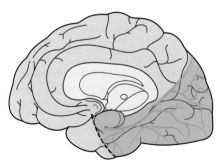

Figure 3.12 **Posterior cerebral artery** The posterior cerebral artery arises from the basilar artery. It supplies the occipital and temporal lobes, midbrain, choroid plexus, thalamus, subthalamic nucleus, optic radiation, corpus callosum and cranial nerves III and IV. The posterior communicating arteries connect the posterior cerebral arteries to the middle cerebral arteries anteriorly.

Signs and symptoms	Structures involved
Thalamic syndrome: hemisensory loss, chorea or hemiballism, spontaneous pain and dysaesthesias	Posterior nucleus of thalamus
Weber's syndrome: oculomotor paralysis and contralateral hemiplegia	Cranial nerve III and cerebral peduncle
Contralateral hemiballism	Subthalamic nucleus
Contralateral homonymous hemianopia	Primary visual cortex or optic radiation
Cortical blindness/cortical visual impairment	Primary visual cortex
Bilateral homonymous hemianopia, visual hallucinations	Bilateral occipital lobe
Alexia, colour anomia, impaired memory, visual agnosia	Dominant corpus callosum (occipital lobe)
Memory defect, amnesia	Bilateral inferomedial portions of temporal lobe
Prosopagnosia	Calcarine sulcus and lingual gyrus (nondominant occipital lobe)

Vertebral and basilar arteries

The vertebral arteries arise from the subclavian arteries at the root of the neck and enter the skull through the foramen magnum. Within the skull they fuse to form the basilar artery. They supply the medulla, pons, midbrain and cerebellum.

Signs and symptoms	Structures involved
Lateral medullary syndrome:	
• vertigo, vomiting, nystagmus	Vestibular nuclei
• ipsilateral limb ataxia	Spinocerebellar tract
• ipsilateral loss of facial pain and thermal sensation	Cranial nerve V
• ipsilateral Horner's syndrome	Descending sympathetic tract

Signs and symptoms	Structures involved
• ipsilateral dysphagia, hoarseness, vocal cord paralysis and reduced gag reflex	Cranial nerves IX and X
• contralateral loss of pain and thermal sensation in trunk and limbs	Lateral spinothalamic tract
Ipsilateral tongue paralysis and hemiatrophy	Cranial nerve XII
Contralateral impaired tactile sensation and proprioception	Medial lemniscus
Diplopia, lateral and vertical gaze palsies, pupillary abnormalities	Cranial nerve VI, medial longitudinal fasciculus
Bulbar palsy, tetraplegia, changes in consciousness	Bilateral corticospinal tracts
Pseudobulbar palsy, emotional instability	Bilateral supranuclear fibres, cranial nerves IX–XII
Locked-in syndrome	Bilateral medulla or pons
Coma, death	Brainstem

Signs and symptoms of injury to the lobes of the brain (adapted from Lindsay et al 2010, with permission)

Frontal lobe

Function	Signs of impairment
Precentral gyrus (motor cortex) Contralateral movement: face, arm, leg, trunk	Contralateral hemiparesis/hemiplegia
Broca's area (dominant hemisphere) Expressive centre for speech	Expressive aphasia (dominant)
Supplementary motor area Contralateral head and eye turning	Paralysis of contralateral head and eye movement

Function	Signs of impairment
Prefrontal areas (damage is often bilateral) 'Personality', initiative	Three prefrontal syndromes are recognized: *Orbitofrontal syndrome* – disinhibition, poor judgement, emotional lability *Frontal convexity syndrome* – apathy, indifference, poor abstract thought *Medial frontal syndrome* – akinetic, incontinent, sparse verbal output Prefrontal lesions are also associated with primitive reflexes (e.g. grasp, pout), disturbance of gait (gait apraxia), resistance to passive movements of the limbs (paratonia)
Paracentral lobule Cortical inhibition of bladder and bowel voiding	Incontinence of urine and faeces

Parietal lobe

Function	Signs of impairment
Postcentral gyrus (sensory cortex) Posture, touch and passive movement	Hemisensory loss/disturbance: postural, passive movement, localization of light touch, two-point discrimination, astereognosis, sensory inattention
Supramarginal and angular gyri *Dominant hemisphere (part of Wernicke's language area):* integration of auditory and visual aspects of comprehension	Receptive aphasia
Nondominant hemisphere: body image, awareness of external environment, ability to construct shapes, etc.	Left-sided inattention, denies hemiparesis Anosognosia, dressing apraxia, geographical agnosia, constructional apraxia

Function	Signs of impairment
Dominant parietal lobe Calculation, using numbers	Finger agnosia, acalculia, agraphia, confusion between right and left
Optic radiation Visual pathways	Homonymous quadrantanopia

Temporal lobe

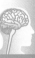

Function	Signs of impairment
Superior temporal gyrus (auditory cortex) Hearing of language (dominant hemisphere), hearing of sounds, rhythm and music (nondominant)	Cortical deafness, difficulty hearing speech – associated with receptive aphasia (dominant), amusia (nondominant), auditory hallucinations
Middle and inferior temporal gyri Learning and memory	Disturbance of memory and learning
Limbic lobe Smell, emotional/affective behaviour	Olfactory hallucinations, aggressive or antisocial behaviour, inability to establish new memories
Optic radiation Visual pathways	Upper homonymous quadrantanopia

Occipital lobe

Function	Signs of impairment
Calcarine sulcus *Primary visual/striate cortex:* Relay of visual information to parastrite cortex	Cortical blindness (bilateral involvement), homonymous hemianopia with or without macular involvement
Association visual/parastriate cortex: Relay of visual information to parietal, temporal and frontal lobes	Cortical blindness without awareness (striate and parastriate involvement), inability to direct gaze associated with agnosia (bilateral parieto-occipital lesions), prosopagnosia (bilateral occipito-temporal lesions)

Signs and symptoms of haemorrhage to other areas of the brain

Putamen

Function	Signs of impairment
Part of basal ganglia Involved in selective movement	Contralateral hemiplegia/hemiparesis, contralateral hemisensory loss, hemianopia (posterior segment), contralateral gaze palsy (posterior segment), receptive-type aphasia (posterior segment, left side), anosognosia (posterior segment, right side), apathy, motor impersistence, temporary unilateral neglect (anterior segment), coma/death (large lesion)

Thalamus

Function	Signs of impairment
Thalamus Receives motor and sensory inputs and transmits them to the cerebral cortex	Contralateral hemiparesis/ hemiplegia, contralateral hemisensory loss, impaired consciousness, ocular disturbances (varied), aphasia (dominant), contralateral neglect (nondominant)

Midbrain

Function	Signs of impairment
Part of brainstem Plays an important role in the control of eye movements and coordination of auditory and visual reflexes. Contains descending motor pathways, ascending sensory pathways, the red nuclei and substantia nigra and cranial nerve nuclei III and IV	Ipsilateral ptosis, dilated pupil, occulomotor nerve weakness, Horner's syndrome. Contralateral hemiparesis including lower face and tongue, contralateral sensory loss including face, contralateral ataxia and intention tremor

Pons

Function	Signs of impairment
Part of brainstem Contains descending motor pathways, ascending sensory pathways and cranial nerve nuclei V–VIII	Coma/death (large bilateral lesions), locked-in syndrome (bilateral), tetraplegia (bilateral), lateral gaze palsy towards affected side, contralateral hemiplegia, contralateral hemisensory loss, ipsilateral facial weakness/sensory loss, ipsilateral ataxia, coarse intention tremor

Cerebellum

Function	Signs of impairment
Anterior lobe (spinocerebellum) Muscle tone, posture and gait control	Hypotonia, postural reflex abnormalities
Posterior lobe (neocerebellum) Coordination of skilled movements	Ipsilateral ataxia: dysmetria, dysdiadochokinesia, intention tremor, rebound phenomenon, dyssynergia, dysarthria
Flocculonodular lobe (vestibulocerebellum) Eye movements and balance	Disturbance of balance, unsteadiness of gait and stance, truncal ataxia, nystagmus, ocular disturbances

Medulla oblongata

Function	Signs of impairment
Part of brainstem Controls breathing, heart and blood vessel function and digestion. Contains descending motor pathways (the lateral corticospinal tract crosses to the contralateral side within the medulla), ascending sensory pathways and the lower cranial nerve nuclei (IX, X, XI, XII)	Contralateral hemiparesis and sensory loss (with sparing of the face). Ipsilateral facial sensory loss (pain and temperature). Ipsilateral Horner's syndrome. Ipsilateral laryngeal, pharyngeal and palatal paralysis (loss of gag reflex) with dysarthria and dysphagia. Ipsilateral ataxia and dysmetria. Nystagmus, nausea, vomiting and vertigo

Functional implications of spinal cord injury

Level	Motor control	Personal independence	Equipment	Mobility
C1–C2	Swallow, talk, chew, blow (cough absent)	Type, turn pages, use telephone and computer	Hoist, respirator, mouthstick, reclining powered wheelchair using breath/chin control	Wheelchair
C3	Neck control, weak shoulder elevation	As above	Hoist, respirator, mouth/head stick, wheelchair as above	Wheelchair
C4	Respiration, neck control, shoulder shrug	Feed possible	Mouth/head stick, hoist, mobile arm supports, wheelchair as above	Wheelchair
C5	Shoulder external rotation, protraction, elbow flexion, supination	Feed, groom, roll in bed, weight shift, push wheelchair on flat, use brake	Adapted feeding/grooming equipment and hand splints, mobile arm supports, powered wheelchair with hand controls or lightweight manual with grips	Wheelchair
C6	Shoulder, elbow flexion, wrist extension, pronation. Weak elbow extension, wrist flexion and thumb control	Tenodesis grip, drink, write, personal ADL, transfers, dress upper body, light domestic chores, push wheelchair on slope	Adapted equipment and splints, transfer board, hand-controlled car, lightweight manual wheelchair; powered for short distances	Bed mobility, bed-to-chair transfers, wheelchair, car

C7	Elbow extension, finger flexion and extension, limited wrist flexion	Dress lower body, personal and skin care, showering, all transfers, pick up from floor, wheelchair sports	Bath board, shower chair, hand-controlled car; wheelchair as above	All transfers, wheelchair, car
C8	Wrist flexion, hand control	Bladder and bowel care	Grab rails, standing frame, nonadapted wheelchair	Stand in frame
T1–T5	Top half of intercostals and long back muscles	Trunk support, improved balance, assisted cough, negotiate kerbs with wheelchair, routine domestic chores	Bilateral knee-ankle orthoses with spinal attachment, standing frame/table	Full wheelchair independence, transfer floor to chair, mobilize with assistance for short distances
T6–T12	Abdominals	Good balance, weak to normal cough, improved stamina	Bilateral knee-ankle orthoses, crutches or frame	Mobilize independently indoors, transfer chair to crutches
L1–L2	Hip flexion		Calipers	Stairs, transfer floor to crutches

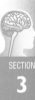

Level	Motor control	Personal independence	Equipment	Mobility
L3–L5	Knee extension, weak knee flexion, dorsiflexion and eversion		Ankle-foot orthoses, crutches/sticks	
S1–S2	Hip extension	Improved standing balance		Normal gait without aids
S2–S4	Bladder, bowel and sexual function			

Autonomic dysreflexia

A potentially life-threatening syndrome that can develop in individuals with a spinal cord lesion at or above T6. It is characterized by an abrupt onset of severe and sustained hypertension. If not treated immediately it can lead to seizures, retinal haemorrhage, pulmonary oedema, myocardial infarction, cerebral haemorrhage and, in some cases, death. Signs include headache, flushed face, bradycardia, sweating above the level of injury, goose bumps below the level of injury, nasal stuffiness and nausea. Autonomic dysreflexia is triggered by a noxious or non-noxious stimulus below the level of the injury. This could be due to irritation of the bladder (urinary tract infection, blocked catheter), bowel (distended or irritated bowel, constipation), skin (cuts, burns, pressure sores, pinching), abdomen (ulcers, gastritis), menstrual cramps or restrictive clothing.

Glossary of neurological terms

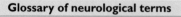

Acalculia	inability to calculate
Agnosia	inability to interpret sensations such as sounds (auditory agnosia), three-dimensional objects by touch (tactile agnosia) or symbols and letters (visual agnosia)
Agraphia	inability to write
Akinesia	loss of the ability to initiate movement and episodes of 'freezing' during movement
Alexia	inability to read
Allodynia	a painful response to a non-noxious stimulus
Amnesia	total or partial loss of memory
Amusia	impaired recognition of music
Aneurysm	a bulge in a blood vessel (usually an artery) caused by a weakness in the vessel wall
Anomia	inability to name objects
Anosmia	loss of ability to smell

Anosognosia	denial of ownership or the existence of a hemiplegic limb
Aphasia	inability to generate and understand language whether verbal or written
Apraxia	a motor planning disorder characterized by an inability to perform learned movements despite intact power, sensation, coordination, perception and understanding. Different forms include ideomotor (inability to carry out motor commands but able to perform movements under different circumstances) and ideational (inability to carry out a sequence of movements, each of which can be performed separately), constructional (inability to build, assemble, or draw objects), occulomotor (impaired voluntary eye movement), dressing and gait.
Astereognosis	inability to recognize objects by touch alone, despite intact sensation
Ataxia	shaky and uncoordinated voluntary movements that may be associated with cerebellar or posterior column disease
Athetosis	involuntary writhing movements affecting face, tongue and hands
Ballismus	sudden, involuntary violent flinging movements of limbs, usually unilateral (hemiballismus)
Bradykinesia	slowness of movement
Bulbar	relating to or involving the medulla oblongata
Chorea	irregular, jerky, involuntary movement
Clonus	more than three rhythmic contractions of the plantarflexors in response to sudden passive dorsiflexion

Decorticate rigidity	characterized by bent arms held in towards the chest, clenched fists and extended lower limbs. Associated with disinhibition of the red nucleus (midbrain) and disruption of the lateral corticospinal tract
Decerebrate rigidity	characterized by extended and internally rotated upper and lower limbs, with the wrists in flexion, the ankles in plantarflexion and the head in extension. Usually indicates damage to the brainstem, specifically lesions in the midbrain and cerebellum
Diplopia	double vision
Dysaesthesia	perverted response to sensory stimuli producing abnormal and sometimes unpleasant sensation
Dysarthria	difficulty articulating speech
Dysdiadochokinesia	clumsiness in performing rapidly alternating movements
Dyskinesia	involuntary movements, e.g. tremor, chorea, dystonia, myoclonus
Dysmetria	under- or overshooting while reaching towards a target
Dysphagia	difficulty or inability to swallow
Dysphasia	difficulty understanding language (receptive dysphasia) or generating language (expressive dysphasia)
Dysphonia	difficulty in producing the voice
Dyssynergia	clumsy, uncoordinated movements
Dystonia	hypertonia associated with abnormal postural movements caused by cocontraction of agonists and antagonists, usually at an extreme of flexion or extension

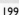

Extrapyramidal signs	refers to the neural network (principally the basal ganglia) located outside the pyramids of the medulla that modulates and regulates pyramidal function (i.e. movement).
Fasciculation	small, local involuntary muscle contraction (twitching)
Graphanaesthesia	inability to recognize numbers or letters traced onto the skin with a blunt object
Hemianopia	loss of one-half of the normal visual field
Hemiparesis	weakness affecting one side of the body
Hemiplegia	paralysis affecting one side of the body
Homonymous	affecting the same side, i.e. homonymous diplopia
Hyperacusis	increased sensitivity to sound
Hyperaesthesia	increased sensitivity to any stimulus
Hyperalgesia	increased sensitivity to a noxious stimulus
Hyperreflexia	increased reflexes
Hypertonia	increase in normal muscle tone
Hypertrophy	abnormal increase in tissue size
Hypoaesthesia	reduced sensitivity to any stimulus
Hypokinesia	slowness in the initiation of movement
Hypotonia	reduced muscle tone
Kinaesthesia	perception of body position and movement
Miosis	pupil constriction
Monoparesis	weakness affecting one limb
Monoplegia	paralysis affecting one limb
Myoclonus	brief, involuntary, shocklike jerks of a muscle/group of muscles
Myotonia	persistent muscle contraction after cessation of voluntary contraction
Nystagmus	involuntary, repetitive, oscillatory movement of the eye in one direction, alternating with a slower movement in the opposite direction
Paraesthesia	tingling sensation often described as 'pins and needles'

Paraphasia	insertion of inappropriate or incorrect words in a person's speech
Paraplegia	paralysis of both legs
Paresis	muscle weakness
Photophobia	intolerance to light
Prosopagnosia	inability to recognize faces
Ptosis	drooping of the upper eyelid
Pyramidal signs	refers to the corticospinal tract that travels from the motor cortex to the brainstem and spinal cord via the pyramids of the medulla. Injuries to the corticospinal tract show characteristics of an upper motor neurone lesion
Rigidity	hypertonia associated with increased resistance to passive stretch that is present at very low speeds of movement, is not velocity-dependent and can affect agonists and antagonists simultaneously and movements in both directions. Subtypes are 'cog-wheel' (increased resistance that gives way in little jerks) and 'lead-pipe' (sustained resistance throughout the whole range of movement).
Quadrantanopia	loss of one-quarter of the normal visual field
Quadraparesis	weakness of all four limbs
Quadriplegia	paralysis of all four limbs
Spasticity	hypertonia associated with exaggerated deep tendon reflexes and a velocity-dependent increase in muscle resistance in response to passive stretch that varies with the direction of joint movement. Subtypes are 'clasp-knife' (initial increased resistance to stretch that suddenly gives way) and 'clonus' (repetitive rhythmic contractions in response to a maintained stretch).

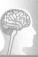

Stereognosis	ability to identify common objects by touch alone
Tetraplegia	another term for quadriplegia
Tetraparesis	another term for quadraparesis

Modified Ashworth scale

Grade	Description
0	Normal tone, no increase in muscle tone
1	Slight increase in muscle tone, manifested by a catch and release or by minimal resistance at the end of the range of motion (ROM) when the affected part(s) is moved in flexion or extension
1+	Slight increase in muscle tone, manifested by a catch, followed by minimal resistance throughout the remainder (less than one-half) of the ROM
2	More marked increase in muscle tone through most of the ROM, but affected part(s) easily moved
3	Considerable increase in muscle tone, passive movement difficult
4	Affected part(s) rigid in flexion or extension

Neurological assessment

Patients present with a variety of conditions, and assessments need to be adapted to suit their needs. This section provides a basic framework for the subjective and objective neurological assessment of a patient.

Database

History of present condition
Past medical history
Drug history
Results of specific investigations (e.g. X-rays, CT scans, blood tests)

Subjective examination

Social situation
- family support
- accommodation
- employment
- leisure activities
- social service support

Normal daily routine
Indoor and outdoor mobility
Personal care (e.g. washing, dressing)
Continence
Vision
Hearing
Swallowing
Fatigue
Pain
Other ongoing treatment
Past physiotherapy and response to treatment
Perceptions of own problems/main concern
Expectations of treatment

Physical examination

Posture and balance

Alignment
Neglect
Sitting balance (static and dynamic)
Standing balance (static and dynamic)
- Romberg's test

Voluntary movement

Range of movement
Strength
Coordination
- finger-nose test
- heel-shin test
- rapidly alternating movement

Endurance

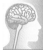

Involuntary movement

Tremor
Clonus
Chorea
Dystonia
Myoclonus
Ballismus
Associated reactions

Tone

Decreased/flaccid
Increased
  * spasticity (clasp-knife or clonus)
  * rigidity (cogwheel or lead-pipe)

Reflexes

Deep tendon reflexes
  * biceps (C5/6)
  * triceps (C7/8)
  * knee (L3/4)
  * ankle (S1/2)
Plantar reflex (Babinski's sign)
Hoffman's reflex

Muscle and joint range

Passive range of movement

Sensory

Light touch
Pin prick
Two-point discrimination
Vibration sense
Joint position sense
Temperature
Vision and hearing

Functional activities

Bed mobility
Sitting balance

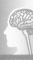

SECTION

3

NEUROLOGY

Transfers
Upper limb function
Mobility
Stairs

Gait

Pattern
Distance
Velocity
Use of walking aids
Orthoses
Assistance from others

Exercise tolerance/fatigue

Cognitive status

Attention
Orientation
Memory

Emotional state

References and Further Reading

Bromley, I. (2006). *Tetraplegia and paraplegia: A guide for physiotherapists* (6th ed.). Edinburgh: Churchill Livingstone.

Davies, P. M. (2000). *Steps to follow: The comprehensive treatment of patients with hemiplegia* (2nd ed.). Berlin: Springer Verlag.

Douglas, G., Nicol, F., & Robertson, C. (2013). *Macleod's clinical examination* (13th ed.). Edinburgh: Churchill Livingstone.

Fuller, G. (2013). *Neurological examination made easy* (5th ed.). Edinburgh: Churchill Livingstone.

Kass, J. S., & Mizrahi, E. M. (2016). *Neurology secrets* (6th ed.). Elsevier.

Lennon, S., & Stokes, M. (2009). *Pocketbook of neurological physiotherapy.* Edinburgh: Churchill Livingstone.

Lindsay, K. W., Bone, I., & Fuller, G. (2010). *Neurology and neurosurgery illustrated* (5th ed.). Edinburgh: Churchill Livingstone.

Mtui, E., Gruener, G., & Dockery, P. (2016). *Fitzgerald's clinical neuroanatomy and neuroscience* (7th ed.). Elsevier.

Ropper, A. H., Samuels, M. A., & Klein, J. P. (2014). *Adams and Victor's principles of neurology* (10th ed.). New York: McGraw-Hill.

Ross, J. (2015). *Crash course: Nervous system* (4th ed.). Edinburgh: Mosby.

Scadding, J. W., & Losseff, N. A. (2011). *Clinical neurology* (4th ed.). CRC Press.

Stokes, M., & Stack, E. (2011). *Physical management for neurological conditions* (3rd ed.). Churchill Livingstone.

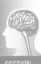

Respiratory

SECTION 4

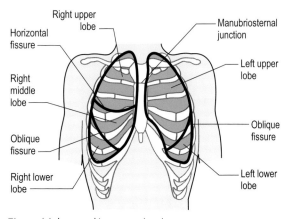

Figure 4.1 Lung markings – anterior view.

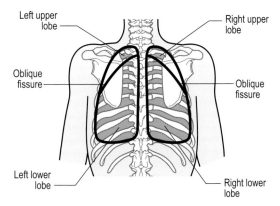

Figure 4.2 Lung markings – posterior view.

Useful lung markings*	
Apex	Anterior – 2.5 cm above medial one-third of clavicles
	Posterior – T1
Inferior border	Anterior – sixth rib
	Posterior – T10/11
	Mid-axilla – eighth rib
Tracheal bifurcation	Anterior – manubriosternal junction
	Posterior – T4
Right horizontal fissure	Anterior – fourth rib (above the nipple)
Oblique fissures	Anterior – sixth rib (below the nipple)
	Posterior – T2/3
Left diaphragm	Anterior – sixth rib
	Posterior – T10
	Mid-axilla – eighth rib
Right diaphragm	Anterior – fifth rib
	Posterior – T9
	Mid-axilla – eighth rib

*These lung markings are approximate and can vary among individuals.

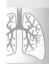

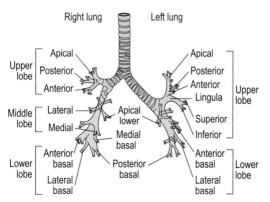

Figure 4.3 Anterior view of brachial tree.

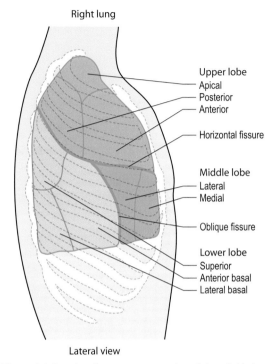

Right lung

Upper lobe
Apical
Posterior
Anterior

Horizontal fissure

Middle lobe
Lateral
Medial

Oblique fissure

Lower lobe
Superior
Anterior basal
Lateral basal

Lateral view

Figure 4.4 Bronchopulmonary segments – lateral view of right lung.

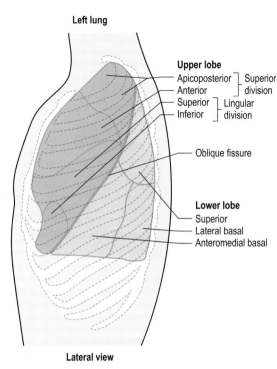

Left lung

Upper lobe
Apicoposterior ⎤ Superior
Anterior ⎦ division
Superior ⎤ Lingular
Inferior ⎦ division

Oblique fissure

Lower lobe
Superior
Lateral basal
Anteromedial basal

Lateral view

Figure 4.5 Bronchopulmonary segments – lateral view of left lung.

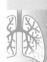

Respiratory volumes and capacities

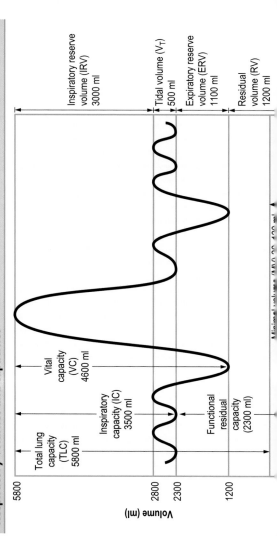

Inspiratory reserve volume (IRV) 3000 ml

Tidal volume (V_T) 500 ml

Expiratory reserve volume (ERV) 1100 ml

Residual volume (RV) 1200 ml

Vital capacity (VC) 4600 ml

Inspiratory capacity (IC) 3500 ml

Functional residual capacity (2300 ml)

Total lung capacity (TLC) 5800 ml

Volume (ml)

5800

2800

2300

1200

Lung volumes

V_T (tidal volume)

Volume of air inhaled or exhaled during a single normal breath
Men: 500 mL   *Women:* 500 mL

IRV (inspiratory reserve volume)

Maximum amount of air that can be inspired on top of a normal tidal inspiration
Men: 3000 mL   *Women:* 1900 mL

ERV (expiratory reserve volume)

Maximum amount of air that can be exhaled following a normal tidal expiration
Men: 1100 mL   *Women:* 700 mL

RV (residual volume)

Volume of air remaining in the lungs after a maximal expiration
Men: 1200 mL   *Women:* 1100 mL

MV (minimal volume)

Amount of air that would remain if the lungs collapsed
Men: 30–120 mL   *Women:* 30–120 mL

Lung capacities

A capacity is the combination of two or more lung volumes.

TLC (total lung capacity)

Total volume of the lungs at the end of a maximal inspiration

$$TLC = VT + IRV + ERV + RV$$

Men: 5800 mL   *Women:* 4200 mL

VC (vital capacity)

Maximum amount of air that can be inspired and expired in a single breath

$$VC = VT + IRV + ERV$$

Men: 4600 mL   *Women:* 3100 mL

IC (inspiratory capacity)

Maximum volume of air that can be inspired after a normal tidal expiration

$$IC = VT + IRV$$

Men: 3500 mL   *Women:* 2400 mL

FRC (functional residual capacity)

Volume of air remaining in the lungs at the end of a normal tidal expiration

$$FRC = ERV + RV$$

Men: 2300 mL   *Women:* 1800 mL

Chest X-rays

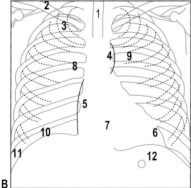

1 Air in the trachea	7 Right ventricle
2 Clavicle	8 Right hilum
3 1st rib	9 Left hilum
4 Aortic arch	10 Right hemidiaphragm
5 Right atrium	11 Costophrenic angle
6 Left ventricle	12 Gastric air bubble

Figure 4.7 **A** Normal posteroanterior chest X-ray. **B** Structures normally visible on X-ray.

Analyzing chest X-rays

Adopt a systematic approach when analyzing X-rays. You should check the following:

Patient's details

* Name, date and time of X-ray

Left and right side

* Ensure that the side marker (left or right) is present and indicates the correct side. The aortic arch, apex of the heart and the gastric air bubble will generally be on the left.

Is it anteroposterior (AP) or posteroanterior (PA)? Supine or erect?

SECTION

4

* AP X-rays are usually taken using a mobile machine with the patient supine. The heart appears larger, and the scapulae overlie the lungs.
* PA X-rays are taken in the radiology department with the patient standing erect. The quality is generally better, and the scapulae are out of the way.
* Vertebral endplates are more visible in AP X-rays and the laminae in PA X-rays.

Is the patient positioned symmetrically?

* The medial ends of the clavicle should be equidistant from the margins or spinous process of the adjacent vertebral body. If the patient is rotated, the position of the heart, spine and rib cage may appear distorted.

Degree of inspiration

* On full inspiration the sixth or seventh rib should intersect the midpoint of the right hemidiaphragm anteriorly or the ninth rib posteriorly.

Exposure

* If the film appears too dark, it is overpenetrated (overexposed).

- If the film appears too light, it is underpenetrated (underexposed).

Think of toast: dark is overdone, and light is underdone.

- The spinous processes of the cervical and upper thoracic vertebra should be visible, as should the outline of the mid-thoracic vertebral bodies.

Extrathoracic soft tissues

- Surgical emphysema is often seen in the supraclavicular areas, around the armpit and the lateral chest wall.
- Note breast shadows in women, which may obscure the lateral wall of the chest.

Invasive medical equipment

- Note the position and presence of any tubes, cannulas, electrodes, etc.
- The tip of the endotracheal tube should lie about 2 cm above the carina.

Bony structures

- Check for fractures, deformities and osteoporosis.

Intercostal spaces

- Small intercostal spaces and steeply sloping ribs indicate reduced lung volume.
- Large intercostal spaces and horizontal ribs indicate hyperinflation.

Trachea

- Lies centrally with the lower one-third inclining slightly to the right.
- Deviation of the trachea indicates mediastinal shift. It shifts towards collapse and away from tumours, pleural effusions and pneumothoraces.
- Bifurcation into the left and right bronchi is normally seen. The right bronchus follows the line of the trachea, whereas the left bronchus branches off at a more acute angle.

Hila

- Composed of the pulmonary vessels and lymph nodes.
- The left and right hilum should be roughly equal in size, though the left hilum appears slightly higher than the right. Their silhouette should be sharp.

Heart

- On a PA film, the diameter of the heart is usually less than one-half the total diameter of the thorax. In the majority of cases, one-third of the cardiac shadow lies on the right and two-thirds on the left, which should be sharply defined. The density of both sides should be equal. The heart may appear larger on an AP film or if the patient is rotated.

Diaphragm

- The right side of the diaphragm is about 2 cm higher than the left because the right lobe of the liver is situated directly underneath it. Both hemidiaphragms should be dome shaped and sharply defined.
- The costophrenic angle is where the diaphragm meets the ribs.
- The cardiophrenic angle is where the diaphragm meets the heart.

Auscultation

Auscultation should be conducted in a systematic manner, comparing the same area on the left and right sides while visualizing the underlying lung structures. Ideally patients should be sitting upright and be asked to breathe through the mouth to reduce nasal turbulence.

Breath sounds
Normal

More prominent at the top of the lungs and centrally, with the volume decreasing towards the bases and periphery. Expiration is shorter and quieter than inspiration and follows inspiration without a pause.

Abnormal (bronchial breathing)

Similar to the breath sounds heard when listening over the trachea. They are typically loud and harsh and can be heard throughout inspiration and expiration. Expiration is longer than inspiration, and there is a pause between the two. They occur if air is replaced by solid tissue, which transmits sound more clearly. Caused by consolidation, areas of collapse with adjacent open bronchus, pleural effusion, tumour.

Diminished

Breath sounds will be reduced if air entry is compromised by either an obstruction or a decrease in airflow. Caused by pneumothorax, pleural effusion, emphysema, collapse with occluded bronchus, atelectasis, inability to breathe deeply, obesity.

Added sounds

Crackles

Heard when airways that have been narrowed or closed, usually by secretions, are suddenly forced open on inspiration. Usually classified as fine (originating from small, distal airways), coarse (from large, proximal airways), localized or widespread. They can be further defined as being early or late, depending on when they are heard on inspiration or expiration.

Early inspiratory – reopening of large airways (e.g. bronchiectasis and bronchitis)
Late inspiratory – reopening of alveoli and peripheral airways (e.g. pulmonary oedema, pulmonary fibrosis, pneumonia, atelectasis)
Early expiratory – secretions in large airways
Late expiratory – secretions in peripheral airways

Wheeze

Caused by air being forced through narrowed or compressed airways. Described as either high or low pitched and monophonic

RESPIRATORY

(single note) or polyphonic (where several airways may be obstructed). Airway narrowing can be caused by bronchospasm, mucosal oedema or sputum retention. An expiratory wheeze with prolonged expiration is usually indicative of bronchospasm, while a low-pitched wheeze throughout inspiration and expiration is normally caused by secretions.

Pleural rub

If the pleural surfaces are inflamed or infected, they become rough and rub together, creating a creaking or grating sound. Heard equally during inspiration and expiration.

Voice sounds

In normal lung tissue, voice sounds are indistinct and unintelligible. When there is consolidation, sound is transmitted more clearly and loudly and speech can be distinguished. Voice sounds can be diminished in the presence of emphysema, pneumothorax and pleural effusion. They can be heard through a stethoscope (vocal resonance) or felt by hand (vocal fremitus). To test voice sounds, patients can be asked to say or whisper '99' repeatedly.

Abnormal breathing patterns

Pursed-lip breathing

Exhalation through tightly drawn lips. This maintains pressure inside the airways, preventing them from collapsing. Often seen in patients with severe airway disease, e.g. COPD.

Paradoxical breathing

This is where normal chest wall movement is reversed. The entire chest wall moves inwards on inspiration and outwards on expiration. Seen in patients with bilateral diaphragm weakness or paralysis, e.g. high cervical spinal cord injury.

Hoover sign

Paradoxical movement of the lower rib cage during inspiration where the lower ribs move inwards instead of outwards. Seen in patients with severe hyperinflation of the lungs where the diaphragm has become flattened and can no longer function as normal.

Kussmaul breathing

A rapid, deep and laboured breathing pattern that is associated with metabolic acidosis, particularly diabetic ketoacidosis and renal failure.

Cheyne-Stokes breathing

Cycles of irregular breathing characterized by a few deep and sometimes rapid breaths followed by gradually shallower breaths often to the point of apnoea. Associated with congestive heart failure, severe neurological insults, e.g. CVA, head injury, brainstem tumours and narcotic or hypnotic drug overdose.

Apneustic breathing

Prolonged inspiration followed by a prominent pause before expiration. Caused by an injury to the brainstem (pons).

Percussion note

Elicited by placing the middle finger of one hand firmly in the space between the ribs and tapping the distal phalanx sharply with the middle finger of the other hand.

The pitch of the note is determined by whether the lungs contain air, solid or fluid and will either sound normal, resonant, dull or stony dull.

Resonant = normal
Hyperresonant = emphysema (bullae) or pneumothorax
Dull = consolidation, areas of collapse, pleural effusion

Sputum analysis (Thomas et al 2016, with permission)

	Description	Causes
Saliva	Clear watery fluid	
Mucoid	Opalescent or white	Chronic bronchitis without infection, asthma

	Description	Causes
Mucopurulent	Slightly discoloured, but not frank pus	Bronchiectasis, cystic fibrosis, pneumonia
Purulent	Thick, viscous: – yellow – dark green/brown – rusty – redcurrant jelly	*Haemophilus* *Pseudomonas* *Pneumococcus, Mycoplasma* *Klebsiella*
Frothy	Pink or white	Pulmonary oedema
Haemoptysis	Ranging from blood specks to frank blood, old blood (dark brown)	Infection (tuberculosis, bronchiectasis), infarction, carcinoma, vasculitis, trauma, also coagulation disorders, cardiac disease
Black	Black specks in mucoid secretions	Smoke inhalation (fires, tobacco, heroin), coal dust

Clubbing

Clubbing is a deformity of the fingernails or toenails in which the angle between the nail bed and nail is lost (the nail-fold or Lovibond's angle). It is usually bilateral, and the distal digital segments can also become enlarged. It is associated with a number of cardiorespiratory and gastrointestinal diseases including lung cancer, bronchiectasis, cystic fibrosis, idiopathic pulmonary fibrosis, congenital heart disease, endocarditis, Crohn's disease, ulcerative colitis and liver disease (primary biliary cirrhosis).

Schamroth's test and window sign

The nail-fold angle is examined by placing the distal phalanx and nail of the same digit of both hands together so that they face each other. Normally, a small diamond-shaped window should appear; however, in digital clubbing this window is obliterated.

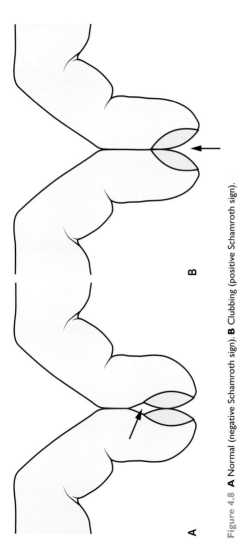

Figure 4.8 **A** Normal (negative Schamroth sign). **B** Clubbing (positive Schamroth sign).

Capillary refill test

A quick test for assessing tissue hydration and blood flow to the peripheral tissues. Position the patient's hand at heart level or above, then apply pressure on the nail bed until it turns white (approximately 5 seconds). Remove the pressure, and measure how long it takes for the colour to return to the nail bed.

Normal capillary refill time is usually less than 2 seconds. A prolonged capillary refill time may be a sign of dehydration or decreased peripheral perfusion, e.g. shock, peripheral vascular disease, hypothermia.

Differential diagnosis of chest pain (data from Thomas et al 2016, with permission)

Pleura (pleurisy)

Causes: pleural infection or inflammation of the pleura, trauma (haemothorax), malignancy
Location: unilateral, often localized
Onset: rapid
Quality: sharp, stabbing
Intensity: often 'catches' at a certain lung volume
Aggravating factors: deep breaths (limits inspiration) and coughing
Relieving factors: anti-inflammatory medication
Associated findings may include: fever, dyspnoea, cough, crackles, pleural rub

Pulmonary embolus

Causes: DVT (secondary to immobilization, long-distance travel)
Location: often lateral, on the side of the embolism but may be central
Onset: sudden
Quality: sharp
Associated findings may include: dyspnoea, tachypnoea, tachycardia, hypotension, hypoxaemia (not significantly improved with oxygen therapy), haemoptysis if

pulmonary infarction occurs. Unilateral swollen lower leg that is red and painful suggests DVT.

Pneumothorax

Causes: trauma, spontaneous, lung diseases (e.g. cystic fibrosis, AIDS), iatrogenic (e.g. post–central line insertion)
Location: Lateral to side of pneumothorax
Onset: sudden
Quality: sharp
Intensity: severity depends on extent of mediastinal shift
Associated findings may include: dyspnea, decreased/absent breath sounds on side of pneumothorax, increased percussion note, tracheal deviation away from the side of the pneumothorax, hypoxaemia

Tracheitis

Causes: bacterial infection (e.g. *Staphylococcus* infection)
Location: central
Quality: burning
Intensity: constant
Aggravating factors: breathing

Tumours

Causes: primary or secondary carcinoma, mesothelioma
Location: may mimic any form of chest pain, depending on site and structures involved
Relieving factors: opiate and anti-inflammatory analgesia

Rib fracture

Causes: trauma, tumour, cough, fractures (e.g. in chronic lung diseases, osteoporosis), iatrogenic (e.g. surgery)
Location: localized point tenderness
Onset: often sudden
Aggravating factors: increases with inspiration

Muscular

Causes: trauma, unaccustomed exercise, excessive coughing during exacerbations of lung disease
Location: superficial

Aggravating factors: increases on inspiration and some body movements

Relieving factors: rest, anti-inflammatory medication, ice or heat

Costochondritis and Tietze syndrome

Causes: trauma, viral infection

Location: localized to one or more costochondral joints

Quality: with or without generalized, nonspecific chest pain

Aggravating factors: sneezing, coughing, deep inspiration, twisting of the chest, reproducible pain – especially at the costochondral junctions

Relieving factors: anti-inflammatory medication, ice or heat

Neuralgia

Causes: thoracic spine dysfunction, tumour, trauma, herpes zoster (shingles)

Location: dermatomal distribution

Quality: sharp or burning or paraesthesia

Relieving factors: antiviral medications (if caused by herpes zoster)

Acute coronary syndrome: angina/myocardial infarction

Causes: ischaemic heart disease

Location: central, retrosternal with or without radiation to the jaw or upper extremities, frequently on left

Onset: pain at rest is more suggestive of infarction

Quality: pressure, tightness, squeezing, heaviness, burning

Aggravating factors: angina is aggravated by exertion, exposure to cold and psychological stress. It usually lasts less than 10 minutes. Myocardial infarction has variable duration but often lasts more than 30 minutes.

Relieving factors: angina is relieved by nitro-glycerine; myocardial infarction is not.

Associated findings: depending on the severity of the ischaemia, they may include nausea, vomiting, dyspnea, dizziness, hypotension, arrhythmias

Pericardium (pericarditis)

Causes: infection, inflammation, trauma, tumour

Location: retrosternal or towards cardiac apex; may radiate to left shoulder

Quality: sharp – may mimic cardiac ischaemia or pleurisy

Relieving factors: may be relieved by sitting up and leaning forwards

Associated findings: tachycardia, pericardial friction rub

Dissecting aortic aneurysm

Causes: trauma, atherosclerosis, Marfan syndrome

Location: anterior chest (often radiating to back, between shoulder blades), poorly localized central chest pain

Onset: sudden onset of unrelenting pain

Quality: tearing or ripping sensation, knifelike

Associated findings: dyspnea, unequal pulses or blood pressure in both arms, hypotension, ischaemic leg pain, reduced lower limb pulses

Oesophageal

Causes: oesophageal reflux, trauma, tumour, vomiting (Boerhaave syndrome)

Location: retrosternal but can also be posterior in the lower back

Quality: burning

Aggravating factors: reflux is aggravated by lying flat or bending forwards after eating

Relieving factors: antacids

Associated findings: oesophageal tears – mediastinal or subcutaneous air or pleural effusion may be seen on CXR

Mediastinal shift

Causes: pneumothorax, rapid drainage of a large pleural effusion

Location: poorly localized, central discomfort

Onset: sudden

Quality: severe

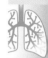

Arterial blood gas analysis

Arterial blood analysis	Reference ranges in adults
pH	7.35–7.45 pH
PaO_2	10.7–13.3 kPa (80–100 mmHg)
$PaCO_2$	4.7–6.0 kPa (35–45 mmHg)
HCO_3^-	22–26 mmol/L
Base excess	−2 to +2

Interpreting acid-base disorders

Assessing acid-base disorders involves examining the pH, $PaCO_2$ and HCO_3^-:

- pH – a low pH (<7.4) indicates a tendency towards acidosis, a high pH (>7.4) indicates a tendency towards alkalosis
- $PaCO_2$ – an increase in $PaCO_2$ leads to acidosis, a decrease to alkalosis
- HCO_3^- – an increase in HCO_3^- leads to alkalosis, a decrease to acidosis

Assessment

$PaCO_2$ is produced by cellular processes and removed by the lungs. An increase or decrease in respiratory function will change the levels of $PaCO_2$.

HCO_3^- is produced by the kidneys. Changes in the ability of the kidneys to produce HCO_3^- or remove hydrogen ions in the body will affect the pH. The renal system reflects changes in metabolic activity within the body.

Establish whether the patient's pH is acidotic, alkalotic or normal.

If the pH is acidotic, establish whether this is due to:

- increased $PaCO_2$ – indicating respiratory acidosis
- decreased HCO_3^- – indicating metabolic acidosis

If the pH is alkalotic, establish whether this is due to:

- decreased $PaCO_2$ – indicating respiratory alkalosis
- increased HCO_3^- – indicating metabolic alkalosis

Compensation

In acid-base disorders, the body tries to maintain haemostasis by bringing the pH back to its normal range. It does this by increasing or decreasing levels of $PaCO_2$ and HCO_3^-. Therefore, if the pH is within normal range, the original abnormality can be identified by comparing the pH to the $PaCO_2$ and the HCO_3^-.

* If the pH is below 7.4 (tending towards acid), then the component that correlates with acidosis (increased $PaCO_2$ or decreased HCO_3^-) is the cause and the other is the compensation.
* If the pH is above 7.4 (tending towards alkaline), the component that correlates with alkalosis (decreased $PaCO_2$ or increased HCO_3^-) is the cause and the other is the compensation.

Simple acid-base disorders

	pH	PaCO$_2$	HCO$_3^-$
Respiratory Acidosis			
Uncompensated	↓	↑	N
Compensated	N	↑	↑
Respiratory Alkalosis			
Uncompensated	↑	↓	N
Compensated	N	↓	↓
Metabolic Acidosis			
Uncompensated	↓	N	↓
Compensated	N	↓	↓
Metabolic Alkalosis			
Uncompensated	↑	N	↑
Compensated	N	↑	↑
↑ = decreased; ↓ = increased; N = normal.			

Base excess

Allows assessment of the metabolic component of acid-base disturbances and therefore the degree of renal compensation that has occurred. A base deficit (less than −2) indicates a metabolic acidosis, and a base excess (greater than +2) correlates with metabolic alkalosis.

Respiratory failure

Broadly defined as an inability of the respiratory system to maintain blood gas values within normal ranges. There are two types:

Type I (hypoxaemic respiratory failure)

A decreased PaO_2 (hypoxaemia) with a normal or slightly reduced $PaCO_2$ due to inadequate gas exchange. Causes include pneumonia, emphysema, fibrosing alveolitis, severe asthma and adult respiratory distress syndrome.
Defined as PaO_2 < 8 kPa (60 mmHg).

Type II (ventilatory failure)

A decreased PaO_2 with an increased $PaCO_2$ (hypercapnia) caused by hypoventilation. Causes include neuromuscular disorders (e.g. muscular dystrophy, Guillain-Barré syndrome), lung diseases (e.g. asthma, COPD), drug-related respiratory drive depression and injuries to the chest wall.
Defined as PaO_2 < 8 kPa (60 mmHg), $PaCO_2$ > 6.7 kPa (50 mmHg).

Arterial blood gas classification of respiratory failure

	pH	$PaCO_2$	HCO_3^-
Acute	↓	↑	N
Chronic	N	↑	↑
Acute on chronic	↓	↑	↑
↓ = decreased; ↑ = increased; N = normal.			

Nasal cannula

The following values are approximate as the patient's flow rates, ability to breathe through the nose, type of cannula and buildup of nasal mucus may all affect the amount of oxygen received. As a general rule, the FiO_2 is raised by 3–4% for each litre of oxygen.

To convert litres of O_2 to FiO_2
RA ≈ 21% FiO_2
1 L/min ≈ 24% FiO_2
2 L/min ≈ 28% FiO_2
3 L/min ≈ 32% FiO_2
4 L/min ≈ 36% FiO_2
5 L/min ≈ 40% FiO_2
6 L/min ≈ 44% FiO_2
RA = room air.

Although nasal cannula may be used with oxygen flows of up to 6 L/min, flow rates above 4 L/min may cause drying and irritation of the nasal mucosa.

Common modes of mechanical ventilation

Continuous mandatory ventilation (CMV)

Delivers a preset number of time-controlled breaths to the patient that can be pressure or volume targeted:

- In volume-targeted CMV (VC-CMV), the ventilator delivers a preset tidal volume and flow rate, with airway pressure being dependent on airflow resistance and compliance of the respiratory system. A pressure limit can be set to limit barotrauma.
- In pressure-targeted CMV (PC-CMV), the ventilator delivers a preset pressure and flow rate, with tidal volume being dependent on airflow resistance and compliance of the respiratory system.
- In dual-control modes (PRVC: pressure-regulated volume control), the ventilator delivers volume-targeted breaths

that are pressure controlled, with peak airway pressure varying from breath to breath, allowing for continuous adaptation to the patient's airway resistance and lung compliance.

The original form of CMV (in which the work of breathing is fully controlled by the ventilator and the patient is unable to breath spontaneously) has been surpassed by newer modes that allow for patient-initiated breaths and can assist or control ventilation dynamically. However, CMV does not allow spontaneous breathing between mandatory breaths.

Intermittent mandatory ventilation (IMV)

Delivers a preset number of time-controlled breaths to the patient that can be pressure or volume targeted but allows the patient to take spontaneous breaths between scheduled machine-delivered breaths. This mode has given way to synchronous intermittent mandatory ventilation (SIMV).

Synchronized intermittent mandatory ventilation (SIMV)

Synchronizes breaths from the ventilator with the patient's spontaneous breaths. If the patient fails to take a spontaneous breath within a set time, the ventilator delivers a mandatory breath that is pressure or volume targeted.

Pressure support (PS)

The patient breathes spontaneously, triggering the ventilator to deliver a set level of positive pressure to assist air entry and reduce the work of breathing. The patient controls the tidal volume, respiratory rate and flow rate. Pressure support can be added to SIMV to compensate for the resistance from the endotracheal tube, making it easier for the patient to breathe.

Complications of mechanical ventilation

Infections, e.g. ventilator-associated pneumonia
Barotrauma, including pneumothorax, interstitial
  emphysema

Tracheal injuries
Ventilator-associated lung injury
Diaphragm atrophy
Oxygen toxicity
Decreased cardiac output

Noninvasive ventilation (NIV)

NIV is the provision of ventilatory support without intubation to the upper airway, usually via a mask or similar device. Positive pressure ventilation is the most common form, though negative pressure ventilation is used in some situations. The most common modes of NIV are CPAP and BiPAP.

Continuous positive airway pressure (CPAP)

A high flow of gas is delivered continuously throughout inspiration and expiration during spontaneous breathing. The alveoli and smaller airways are splinted open, increasing lung volume at the end of expiration (i.e. the functional residual capacity). The aim is to reverse atelectasis and improve gas exchange. It also increases lung compliance and decreases the work of breathing.

Bilevel positive airway pressure (BiPAP)

Similar to CPAP, positive airway pressure is delivered throughout inspiration and expiration during spontaneous breathing, but the level of positive airway pressure alters between inspiration and expiration. A higher level is delivered during inspiration and a lower level during expiration. The alteration between pressure levels is synchronized with the patient's breathing.

Contraindications to NIV

- Facial trauma/burns
- Recent facial, upper airway or upper gastrointestinal tract surgery
- Fixed obstruction of the upper airway
- Inability to protect airway
- Life-threatening hypoxaemia

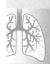

- Haemodynamic instability requiring inotropes/pressors (unless in a critical care unit)
- Severe comorbidity
- Confusion/agitation
- Vomiting
- Bowel obstruction
- Copious respiratory secretions
- Undrained pneumothorax

Cardiorespiratory monitoring

Arterial blood pressure (ABP)

Measured via an intra-arterial cannula which allows continuous monitoring of the patient's blood pressure and also provides an access for arterial blood sampling and blood gas analysis.

Normal value: 95/60–140/90 mmHg in adults (increases gradually with age)
Hypertension: >145/95 mmHg
Hypotension: <90/60 mmHg

Cardiac output (CO)

Amount of blood pumped into the aorta each minute.

$$CO = HR \times SV$$

Normal value: 4–8 L/min

Cardiac index (CI)

Cardiac output related to body size. Body surface area is calculated by using the patient's weight and height and a nomogram. Allows reliable comparison between patients of different sizes.

$$CI = CO \div \text{body surface area}$$

Normal value: 2.5–4 L/min/m^2

Central venous pressure (CVP)

Measured via a central venous cannula inserted into the internal or external jugular vein or subclavian vein with the tip resting close to the right atrium within the superior vena cava. Provides information on circulating blood volume, the effectiveness of the heart to pump that volume, vascular tone and venous return.

Normal value: 3–15 cmH$_2$O

Cerebral perfusion pressure (CPP)

Pressure required to ensure adequate blood supply to the brain.

$$CPP = MAP - ICP$$

Normal value: >70 mmHg

Ejection fraction (EF)

The stroke volume (SV) as a percentage of the total volume of the ventricle prior to systolic contraction, i.e. end-diastolic volume (EDV).

$$EF = SV \div EDV$$

Normal value: 65–75%

Heart rate (HR)

The number of times the heart contracts in 1 minute.

Normal value: 50–100 beats/min
Tachycardia: >100 beats/min at rest
Bradycardia: <50 beats/min at rest

Intracranial pressure (ICP)

Pressure exerted by the brain tissue, cerebrospinal fluid and blood volume within the rigid skull and meninges. Neurological insults such as space-occupying lesions, cerebral oedema, hydrocephalus, cerebral haemorrhage, hypoxia and infection cause this pressure to rise, resulting in a decreased blood supply to the brain. When treating patients with raised ICP, minimize handling and ensure that the head is maintained in midline and raised 15–30° from supine. A marked degree of hip flexion should be avoided to ensure optimal circulation and prevent potential increase in ICP.

Normal value: 0–10 mmHg

Mean arterial pressure (MAP)

Measures the average pressure of blood being pushed through the circulatory system. It relates to cardiac output and systemic vascular resistance and reflects tissue perfusion pressure.

$$MAP = (diastolic\ BP \times 2) + (systolic\ BP) \div 3$$

Normal value: 80–100 mmHg
<60 mmHg indicates inadequate circulation to the vital organs

Oxygen saturation (SpO$_2$)

Arterial oxygen saturation is measured using noninvasive pulse oximetry.

Normal value: 95–98%

Pulmonary artery pressure (PAP)

A pulmonary artery balloon catheter (Swan-Ganz) is inserted via the CVP catheter route and floated into the pulmonary artery via the right ventricle. The PAP measures pressures of the blood in the vena cava, right atrium and right ventricle and provides a measure of the ability of the right side of the heart to push blood through the lungs and to the left side of the heart.

Normal value: 15–25/8–15 mmHg
Mean value: 10–20 mmHg

Pulmonary artery occlusion pressure (PAOP)

Similar to PAP, but the Swan-Ganz catheter is moved further along until it wedges in a small pulmonary artery. The balloon tip is inflated to occlude the artery in order to allow measurement of the pressure in the pulmonary capillaries in front of it and the left atrium. Previously know as pulmonary artery wedge pressure (PAWP).

Normal value: 6–12 mmHg

Respiratory rate (RR)

Number of breaths taken in 1 minute.

Normal value: 12–16 breaths/min
Tachypnoea: >20 breaths/min
Bradypnoea: <10 breaths/min

Stroke volume (SV)

The amount of blood ejected from the ventricles during each systolic contraction. Affected by preload (amount of tension on the ventricular wall before it contracts), afterload (resistance that the ventricle must work against when it contracts) and contractility (force of contraction generated by the myocardium).

$$SV = (CO \times 1000) \div HR$$

Normal value: 60–130 mL/beat

Systemic vascular resistance (SVR)

Evaluates the vascular component of afterload in the left ventricle. Vasoconstriction will increase systemic vascular resistance, whereas vasodilation will decrease it.

$$SVR = 80 \times (MAP - CVP) \div CO$$

Normal value: 800–1400 dyn · s · cm^{-5}

ECGs

ECGs detect the sequence of electrical events that occur during the contraction (depolarization) and relaxation (repolarization) cycle of the heart. Depolarization is initiated by the sinoatrial (SA) node, the heart's natural pacemaker, which transmits the electrical stimulus to the atrioventricular (AV) node. From here, the impulse is conducted through the bundle of His and along

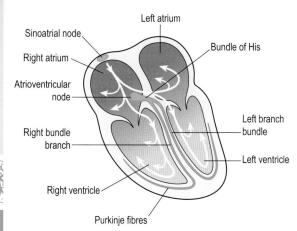

Left atrium

Sinoatrial node

Bundle of His

Right atrium

Atrioventricular node

Left branch bundle

Right bundle branch

Left ventricle

Right ventricle

Purkinje fibres

Figure 4.9 Conduction system of the heart.

the bundle branches to the Purkinje fibres, causing the heart to contract.

The atrioventricular (AV) node can also function as a pacemaker when there is a dysfunction of the SA node, e.g. failure to generate an impulse (sinus arrest), when the impulse generated is too slow (sinus bradycardia) or when the impulse is not conducted to the AV node (SA block, AV block).

ECGs are recorded on graphed paper that travels at 25 mm/s. It is divided into large squares of 5-mm width, which represents 0.2 s horizontally. Each square is then divided into five squares of 1 mm width (i.e. 0.04 s horizontally). Electrical activity is measured in millivolts (mV). A 1 mV signal moves the recording stylus vertically 1 cm (i.e. two large squares).

An ECG complex consists of five waveforms labelled with the letters P, Q, R, S and T, which represent the electrical events that occur in one cardiac cycle.

The P wave represents the activation of the atria (atrial depolarization).

- P amplitude: <2.5 mm
- P duration: 0.06–0.12 s

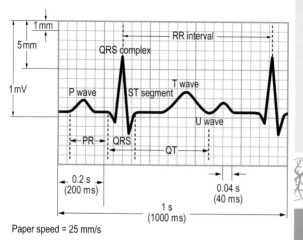

Paper speed = 25 mm/s

Figure 4.10 Normal ECG.

The PR interval represents the time between the onset of atrial depolarization and the onset of ventricular depolarization, i.e. the time taken for the impulse to travel from the SA node through the AV node and the His-Purkinje system.

- PR duration: 0.12–0.20s

The QRS complex represents the activation of the ventricles (ventricular depolarization).

- QRS amplitude: 5–30 mm
- QRS duration: 0.06–0.10s

The ST segment represents the end of ventricular depolarization and the beginning of ventricular repolarization.

The T wave represents ventricular repolarization.

- T amplitude: <10 mm (approximately more than one-eighth but less than two-thirds of corresponding R wave)

The QT interval represents the total time for ventricular depolarization and repolarization.

- QT duration: 0.35–0.45 s

The U wave represents repolarization of the His-Purkinje system and is not always present on an ECG.

Examples of ECGs

Normal sinus rhythm

* Regular rhythms and rates (60–100 beats/min)
* Has a P wave, QRS complex and T wave; all similar in size and shape

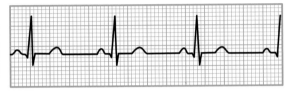

Figure 4.11 Sinus rhythm.

Sinus bradycardia

Defined as a sinus rhythm with a resting heart rate of less than 60 beats/min.

* Heart rate <60 beats/min
* Regular sinus rhythm

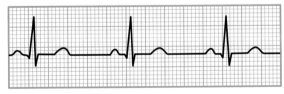

Figure 4.12 Sinus bradycardia.

Causes include cardiomyopathy, acute myocardial infarction, drugs (e.g. β blockers, digoxin, amiodarone), obstructive jaundice, raised intracranial pressure, sick sinus syndrome, hypothermia, hypothyroidism, electrolyte abnormalities.

Can be a normal finding in extremely fit individuals and during sleep.

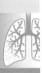

Sinus tachycardia

Defined as a sinus rhythm with a resting heart rate of more than 100 beats/min.

- Heart rate >100 beats/min
- Regular sinus rhythm

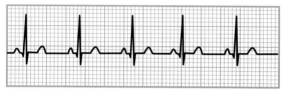

Figure 4.13 Sinus tachycardia.

Causes include sepsis, fever, anaemia, pulmonary embolism, hypovolaemia, hypoxia, hyperthyroidism, phaeochromocytoma, drugs (e.g. salbutamol, alcohol, caffeine).

Can occur as a response to increased demand for blood flow, e.g. exercise or in high emotional states, e.g. fear, anxiety, pain.

Atrial fibrillation

Where rapid, unsynchronized electrical activity is generated in the atrial tissue, causing the atria to quiver. Transmission of the impulses to the ventricles via the AV node is variable and unpredictable, leading to an irregular heartbeat.

- Absent P wave replaced by fine baseline oscillations (atrial impulses fire at a frequency of 350–600 beats/min)
- Irregular ventricular complexes; RR interval irregular
- Ventricular rate varies between 100 and 180 beats/min but can be slower

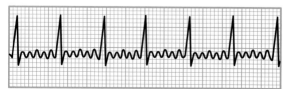

Figure 4.14 Atrial fibrillation.

Causes include hypertension, coronary artery disease, mitral valve disease, post–cardiac surgery, sick sinus syndrome, pneumonia, pulmonary embolism, hyperthyroidism, alcohol misuse, chronic pulmonary disease.

Ventricular ectopics or premature ventricular contractions (PVCs)

Early beats (ectopics) usually caused by electrical irritability in the ventricular conduction system or myocardium. Can occur in normal individuals and be asymptomatic. However, can indicate impending fatal arrhythmias in patients with heart disease. Can occur singly, in clusters of two or more or in repeating patterns such as bigeminy (every other beat) or trigeminy (every third beat).

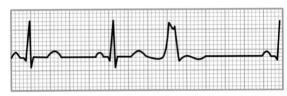

Figure 4.15 Ventricular ectopics and PVCs.

- Irregular rhythm during PVC; however, underlying rhythm and rate is usually regular, i.e. sinus
- P wave absent, QRS complex wide and early, T wave in opposite direction from QRS complex during PVC

Causes include acute myocardial infarction; valvular heart disease; electrolyte disturbances; metabolic acidosis; medications including digoxin and tricyclic antidepressants; drugs such as cocaine, amphetamines and alcohol; anaesthetics and stress.

Ventricular tachycardia

Defined as three or more heartbeats of ventricular origin at a rate exceeding 100 beats/minute. May occur in short bursts of less than 30 seconds, and may terminate spontaneously with few or no symptoms (nonsustained). Episodes lasting more than

30 seconds (sustained) lead to rapid deterioration and ventricular fibrillation that requires immediate treatment to prevent death.

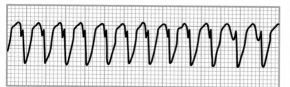

Figure 4.16 Ventricular tachycardia.

* Ventricular rate 100–200 beats/min
* Ventricular rhythm is usually regular
* QRS complex is wide, P wave is absent

Causes include acute myocardial infarction, myocardial ischaemia, cardiomyopathy, mitral valve prolapse, electrolyte imbalance, drugs (digoxin, antiarrhythmics), myocarditis.

Ventricular fibrillation

Rapid, ineffective contractions of the ventricles caused by chaotic electrical impulses resulting in no cardiac output. Unless treated immediately, it is fatal.

Ventricular fibrillation is the most commonly identified arrhythmia in cardiac arrest patients and the primary cause of sudden cardiac death (SCD).

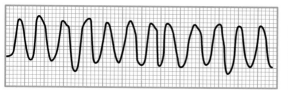

Figure 4.17 Ventricular fibrillation.

No recognizable pattern: irregular, chaotic, immeasurable.

Biochemical and haematological studies

Blood serum studies

Test	Function	Interpretation
Albumin 36–47 g/L	Most abundant plasma protein. Maintains osmotic pressure of the blood. Transports blood constituents such as fatty acids, hormones, enzymes, drugs and other substances	*Increased:* relative increase with haemoconcentration, where there is severe loss of body water *Decreased:* malnutrition, malabsorption, severe liver disease, renal disease, gastrointestinal conditions causing excessive loss, thyrotoxicosis, chemotherapy, Cushing's disease
Bilirubin 2–17 mmol/L	Pigment produced by the breakdown of haem	*Increased:* hepatitis, biliary tract obstruction, haemolysis, haematoma *Decreased:* iron-deficiency anaemia
C-reactive protein <7 mg/L	Protein produced in the acute inflammatory phase of injury. Index for monitoring disease activity	*Increased:* pyrexia, all inflammatory conditions (e.g. rheumatoid arthritis, pneumococcal pneumonia), trauma, during late pregnancy

Calcium 2.1–2.6 mmol/L	Nerve impulse transmission, bone and teeth formation, skeletal and myocardial muscle contraction, activation of enzymes, blood coagulation, cell division and repair, membrane structure and absorption of vitamin B_{12}	*Increased (hypercalcaemia):* hyperparathyroidism, malignancy, Paget's disease, osteoporosis, immobilization, renal failure *Decreased (hypocalcaemia):* hypoparathyroidism, vitamin D deficiency, acute pancreatitis, low blood albumin, low blood magnesium, large transfusion of citrated blood, increased urine excretion, respiratory acidosis
Creatine kinase Men: 30–200 U/L Women: 30–150 U/L	Enzyme found in heart, brain and skeletal muscle. Increased when one of these areas is stressed or damaged. Testing for a specific creatine kinase isoenzyme indicates area of damage (e.g. raised CK-MB indicates damage to heart)	*Increased:* heart (myocardial infarction, myocarditis, open heart surgery), brain (brain cancer, trauma, seizure) and skeletal muscle damage (intramuscular injections, trauma, surgery, strenuous exercise, muscular dystrophy)
Creatinine 55–150 mmol/L	End-product of normal muscle metabolism	*Increased:* renal failure, urinary obstruction, muscle disease *Decreased:* pregnancy, muscle wasting
Glucose 3.6–5.8 mmol/L	Metabolized in the cells to produce energy	*Increased:* diabetes mellitus, Cushing's disease, patients on steroid therapy *Decreased:* severe liver disease, adrenocortical insufficiency, drug toxicity, digestive diseases

Test	Function	Interpretation
Lactate dehydrogenase 230–460 U/L	Enzyme that converts pyruvic acid into lactate. High levels found in myocardial and skeletal muscle, the liver, lungs, kidneys and red blood cells	*Increased:* tissue damage due to myocardial infarction, liver disease, renal disease, cellular damage in trauma, hypothyroidism, muscular diseases
Magnesium 0.7–1.0 mmol/L	Neuromuscular transmission, cofactor in activation of many enzyme systems for cellular metabolism (e.g. phosphorylation of glucose, production and functioning of ATP), regulation of protein synthesis	*Increased (hypermagnesaemia):* renal failure, adrenal insufficiency, excessive oral or parenteral intake of magnesium, severe dehydration
		Decreased (hypomagnesaemia): excessive loss from gastrointestinal tract (diarrhoea, nasogastric suction, pancreatitis), decreased gut absorption, renal disease, long-term use of certain drugs (e.g. diuretics, digoxin), chronic alcoholism, increased aldosterone secretion, polyuria
Phosphate 0.8–1.4 mmol/L	Bone formation, formation of high energy compounds (e.g. ATP), nucleic acid synthesis, enzyme activation	*Increased (hyperphosphataemia):* renal failure, hypoparathyroidism, chemotherapy, excessive phosphorus intake
		Decreased (hypophosphataemia): hyperparathyroidism, chronic alcoholism, diabetes, respiratory alkalosis, excessive glucose ingestion, hypoalimentation, chronic use of antacids

Potassium 3.6–5.0 mmol/L	Nerve impulse transmission, contractility of myocardial, skeletal and smooth muscle	*Increased (hyperkalaemia):* renal failure, increased intake of potassium, metabolic acidosis, tissue trauma (e.g. burns and infection), potassium-sparing diuretics, adrenal insufficiency *Decreased (hypokalaemia):* potassium-wasting diuretics, vomiting, diarrhoea, metabolic alkalosis, excess aldosterone secretion, polyuria, profuse sweating
Sodium 136–145 mmol/L	Regulates body's water balance, maintains acid-base balance and electrical nerve potentials	*Increased (hypernatraemia):* excessive fluid loss or salt intake, water deprivation, diabetes insipidus, excess aldosterone secretion, diarrhoea *Decreased (hyponatraemia):* kidney disease, excessive water intake, adrenal insufficiency, diarrhoea, profuse sweating, diuretics, congestive heart failure, inappropriate secretion of ADH
Urea 2.5–6.5 mmol/L	Waste product of metabolism	*Increased:* renal failure, decreased renal perfusion because of heart disease, shock *Decreased:* high-carbohydrate/low-protein diets, late pregnancy, malabsorption, severe liver damage

Haematological studies

Test	Assesses	Interpretation
Red blood cell count (RBC) *Men:* $4.5–6.5 \times 10^{12}$/L *Women:* $3.8–5.3 \times 10^{12}$/L	Blood loss, anaemia, polycythaemia (increase in Hb concentration of the blood)	*Increased:* polycythaemia vera, dehydration, cardiac and pulmonary disorders characterized by cyanosis, acute poisoning *Decreased:* leukaemia, anaemia, fluid overload, haemorrhage
White blood cell count (WBC) $4.0–11.0 \times 10^{9}$/L	Detects infection or inflammation. Monitors response to radiation and chemotherapy	*Increased:* leukaemia, tissue necrosis, infection *Decreased:* bone marrow suppression
White blood cell differential *Neutrophils:* $1.5–7.0 \times 10^{9}$/L *Eosinophils:* $0.0–0.4 \times 10^{9}$/L *Lymphocytes:* $1.2–3.5 \times 10^{9}$/L *Monocytes:* $0.2–1.0 \times 10^{9}$/L *Basophils:* $0.0–0.2 \times 10^{9}$/L	Evaluates body's ability to resist infection. Detects and classifies leukaemia	*Increased:* Neutrophil – bacterial infection, noninfective acute inflammation, tissue damage Eosinophil – allergic reaction, parasitic worm infection Lymphocyte – viral infection, chronic bacterial infection Monocyte – chronic bacterial infection, malignancy Basophil – myeloproliferative disorders

Packed cell volume (PCV)/haematocrit (Hct) *Men:* 0.40–0.54 L/L *Women:* 0.35–0.47 L/L	Blood loss and fluid balance	*Increased:* polycythaemia, dehydration *Decreased:* anaemia, acute blood loss, haemodilution
Haemoglobin (Hb) *Men:* 130–180 g/L *Women:* 115–165 g/L	Anaemia and polycythaemia	*Increased:* polycythaemia, dehydration *Decreased:* anaemia, recent haemorrhage, fluid overload
Platelets (Plt) $150–100 × 10^9/L$	Severity of thrombocytopenia	*Increased:* polycythaemia vera, splenectomy, malignancy *Decreased:* anaemias, infiltrative bone marrow disease, haemolytic disorders, disseminated intravascular coagulopathy, idiopathic thrombocytopenic purpura, viral infections, AIDS, splenomegaly, with radiation or chemotherapy
Prothrombin time (PT) 12–16 s	Measures extrinsic clotting time of blood plasma and clotting factor deficiencies	*Increased:* bile duct obstruction, liver disease, disseminated intravascular coagulation, malabsorption of nutrients from gastrointestinal tract, vitamin K deficiency, warfarin therapy, factor I (fibrinogen), II (prothrombin), V, VII, X deficiency

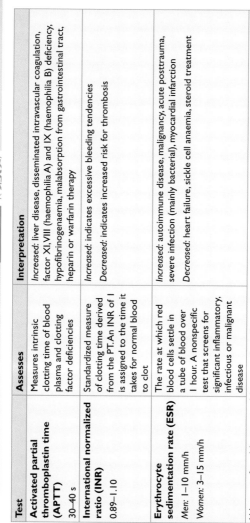

Test	Assesses	Interpretation
Activated partial thromboplastin time (APTT) 30–40 s	Measures intrinsic clotting time of blood plasma and clotting factor deficiencies	*Increased:* liver disease, disseminated intravascular coagulation, factor XI, VIII (haemophilia A) and IX (haemophilia B) deficiency, hypofibrinogenaemia, malabsorption from gastrointestinal tract, heparin or warfarin therapy
International normalized ratio (INR) 0.89–1.10	Standardized measure of clotting time derived from the PT. An INR of 1 is assigned to the time it takes for normal blood to clot	*Increased:* indicates excessive bleeding tendencies *Decreased:* indicates increased risk for thrombosis
Erythrocyte sedimentation rate (ESR) *Men:* 1–10 mm/h *Women:* 3–15 mm/h	The rate at which red blood cells settle in a tube of blood over 1 hour. A nonspecific test that screens for significant inflammatory, infectious or malignant disease	*Increased:* autoimmune disease, malignancy, acute posttrauma, severe infection (mainly bacterial), myocardial infarction *Decreased:* heart failure, sickle cell anaemia, steroid treatment

Values vary from laboratory to laboratory, depending on testing methods used. These reference ranges should be used as a guide only. All reference ranges apply to adults only; they may differ in children.

Data from Matassarin-Jacobs, with permission of WB Saunders

Treatment techniques

Positioning

Adult

Positioning the patient optimizes cardiovascular and cardio-pulmonary function and thus oxygen transport. Correct positioning of the patient can maximize lung volume, lung compliance and the ventilation/perfusion ratio. It can also reduce the work of breathing and aid secretion removal and cough. This may involve positioning adult patients with unilateral lung disease in side lying with the affected lung uppermost to gain the greatest benefit. The situation is reversed in ventilated adult patients, when it is more beneficial for the unaffected lung to be uppermost.

Children and infants

Positioning small children and infants to maximize ventilation/perfusion – rather than for postural drainage and removal of secretions – requires a different approach to adults. In nonventilated children with unilateral lung disease, the unaffected lung should be positioned uppermost. Conversely, ventilated babies and small children should be positioned with the affected lung uppermost to improve oxygenation.

Postural drainage

Positioning the patient according to the anatomy of the bronchial tree in order to use gravity to assist drainage of secretions.

Contraindications and precautions for head-down position (Harden et al 2009, with permission)

- Hypertension
- Severe dyspnoea
- Recent surgery
- Severe haemoptysis
- Nosebleeds
- Advanced pregnancy
- Hiatus hernia

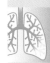

- Cardiac failure
- Cerebral oedema
- Aortic aneurysm
- Head or neck trauma/surgery
- Mechanical ventilation

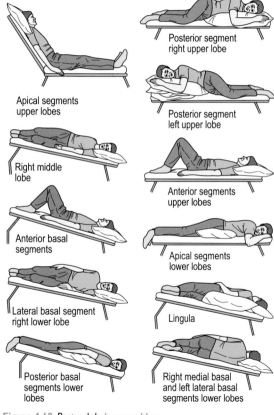

Figure 4.18 Postural drainage positions.

Diaphragmatic paralysis/weakness (adults)

Head-down position can cause reflux, vomiting and
aspiration, and splints the diaphragm reducing respiratory
effectiveness (child/baby)

Manual chest clearance techniques

These can be used while the patient is in a postural drainage
position to aid the clearance of secretions. Manual techniques
include percussion, vibrations and shaking.

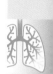

	Contraindications	Precautions
Percussion *Rhythmic clapping with cupped hands or soft-rimmed face mask (in babies) on the patient's chest*	Directly over rib fracture Directly over surgical incision or graft Frank haemoptysis Severe osteoporosis Hypoxia in children and babies – percussion can exacerbate hypoxia, especially in infants	Profound hypoxaemia Bronchospasm Pain Osteoporosis Bony metastases Near chest drains Ensure baby's head is supported
Vibrations *Fine oscillations applied to the chest wall by the therapist's hands or fingertips (in babies). Performed during thoracic expansion exercises, on exhalation only*	Directly over rib fracture Directly over surgical incision Severe bronchospasm Premature infants – causes brain injury if head is not supported	Long-term oral steroids Osteoporosis Near chest drains Rib fractures in children/babies Ensure head is supported in children/babies

SECTION

4

RESPIRATORY

	Contraindications	Precautions
Shaking *Coarse oscillations by compressing and releasing the chest wall. Performed during thoracic expansion exercises, on exhalation only*	Directly over rib fracture Directly over surgical incision Premature infants – causes brain injury. DO NOT USE.	Long-term oral steroids Osteoporosis Bony metastases Near chest drains Severe bronchospasm Rib fractures in children/babies Ensure head is supported in children/babies

From Harden et al 2009, with permission.

Active cycle of breathing technique (ACBT)

This consists of three different breathing techniques, namely breathing control (normal tidal breaths), thoracic expansion exercises (deep inspiratory breaths, usually combined with a 3-s end-inspiratory hold) and forced expiration technique (forced expirations following a breath in that can be performed at different lung volumes), that are repeated in cycles in order to mobilize and clear bronchial secretions. These can be used in different combinations according to the patient's needs and in conjunction with other treatment techniques.

Contraindications

- None if technique(s) adapted to suit the patient's condition

Precautions

- Bronchospasm

Airway suction

The removal of bronchial secretions through a suction catheter inserted via the nose (nasopharyngeal/NP) or mouth (oropharyngeal), or via a tracheostomy or endotracheal tube using vacuum pressure (usually in the range 8.0–20 kPa/60–150 mmHg).

Contraindications

- CSF leak/basal skull fracture (applies to nasopharyngeal approach only)
- Stridor
- Severe bronchospasm
- Acute pulmonary oedema

Precautions

- Severe CVS instability
- Anticoagulated patients or those with clotting disorders
- Recent oesophagectomy, lung transplant or pneumonectomy

Adverse effects

- Tracheobronchial trauma
- Bronchospasm
- Atelectasis
- Pneumothorax
- Hypoxia
- Cardiac arrhythmias
- Raised ICP

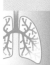

Manual hyperinflation (MHI)

The use of a rebreathing bag to manually inflate the lungs in order to improve lung volume and arterial oxygenation, aid the removal of secretions and assess or improve lung compliance. The peak airway pressure being delivered should not exceed 40 cmH_2O.

Contraindications

- Undrained pneumothorax
- Bullae
- Surgical emphysema
- Cardiovascular instability/arrhythmias
- Patients at risk for barotrauma, e.g. emphysema, fibrosis
- Recent pneumonectomy/lobectomy (first 10 days)
- Severe bronchospasm

- Peak airway pressure >40 cmH$_2$O when mechanically ventilated
- High PEEP requirement >15 cm H$_2$O. If PEEP requirement >10 cm H$_2$O, only use MHI if essential
- Unexplained haemoptysis
- Increased ICP above the set limits

Adverse effects

- Barotrauma
- Haemodynamic compromise – reduced or increased blood pressure
- Cardiac arrhythmia
- Reduced oxygen saturation
- Raised intracranial pressure
- Reduced respiratory drive
- Bronchospasm

Considerations when treating patients with raised ICP
Minimize suction
Minimize manual techniques
Minimize manual hyperinflation (maintain hypocapnia)
Consider sedation/inotropic support if ICP increased or unstable
Monitor CPP: should be >70 mmHg

Intermittent positive pressure breathing (IPPB)

Assisted breathing using positive airway pressure to deliver gas throughout inspiration until a preset pressure is reached. Inspiration is triggered when the patient inhales and expiration is passive.

Effects

- Increases tidal volume
- Reduces work of breathing
- Assists clearance of bronchial secretions
- Improves alveolar ventilation

Contraindications

IPPB should not normally be used when any of the following conditions are present. If in doubt, medical advice should be sought.

- Undrained pneumothorax
- Facial fractures
- Acute head injury
- Large bullae
- Lung abscess
- Severe haemoptysis
- Vomiting
- Cardiovascular instability
- Active tuberculosis
- Tumour or obstruction in proximal airways
- Surgical emphysema
- Recent lung and oesophageal surgery

Tracheostomies

A tracheostomy is an opening in the anterior wall of the trachea to facilitate ventilation. It is sited below the level of the vocal cords.

Indications

- Provide and maintain a patent airway when the upper airways are obstructed.
- Provide access for the removal of tracheobronchial secretions.
- Prevent aspiration of oral and gastric secretions in patients who are unable to protect their own airways.
- Used in patients who need longer-term ventilation.

Types of tube
Metal or plastic

- Metal tubes are used for long-term tracheostomy patients as they are more durable, inhibit bacteria growth, are easier to clean and can be sterilized with heat or steam.

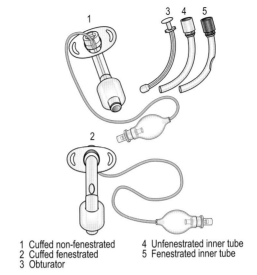

1 Cuffed non-fenestrated   4 Unfenestrated inner tube
2 Cuffed fenestrated   5 Fenestrated inner tube
3 Obturator

Figure 4.19 Different types of tracheostomy tubes.

They are made of either stainless steel or sterling silver
and do not have connections for respiratory equipment,
e.g. a resuscitation bag. On some tubes an adaptor can be
attached.

- Plastic tubes are cheaper and therefore more disposable.

Cuffed or uncuffed

- Cuffed tubes have an air-filled sac at their distal end.
When inflated, a cuffed tube provides a seal between the
trachea and the tube. It protects the airway against
aspiration and allows positive pressure ventilation.
Patients cannot speak when the cuff is inflated, unless the
tube is fenestrated. To minimize the risk for tracheal wall
trauma or aspiration, the cuff pressure should be
regularly checked and maintained between 20 and

30 cmH$_2$O (22 mmHg) or within locally agreed protocols.

- Uncuffed tubes are suitable for long-term use in patients who may still require suctioning to clear secretions. It is essential that patients are able to protect their own airways and have an effective cough and gag reflex to prevent aspiration. In the event of a tracheostomy becoming blocked, the patient may still be able to breathe around the tube. There is less risk for tracheal damage, and the tube is easier to replace.

Fenestrated

- Fenestrated tubes have an opening on the outer cannula. This enables air to pass through the tube and over the vocal cords, allowing speech. They can also be used as part of the weaning process by allowing patients to breathe through the tube and use their upper airways.

Single or double lumen

- Single-lumen tubes consist of a single cannula and are used for invasive ventilation. They are for short-term use only as they carry the risk of becoming blocked by secretions and obstructing the airway. The advantage of using a single lumen is that it maximizes the size of the tube thereby decreasing airway resistance.
- Double-lumen tubes consist of an inner and outer cannula. The inner cannula is removable and can be cleaned to prevent the accumulation of secretions. To allow speech, the inner tube and outer tube need to be fenestrated. However, during suctioning the inner tube must be replaced with an unfenestrated tube to prevent the catheter passing through the fenestration. It must also be in place if the patient is put on positive pressure ventilation in order to maintain pressure.

Mini tracheostomy

- A small tracheostomy that is primarily indicated for sputum retention as it allows regular suctioning. It does not prevent aspiration and will only provide a route for oxygenation in an emergency situation. Talking and swallowing are unaffected.

Complications

- Haemorrhage
- Pneumothorax
- Tracheal tube misplacement
- End of tube blocked if pressed against carina or tracheal wall
- Surgical emphysema
- Secretions occluding tube
- Herniation of cuff causing tube blockage
- Stenosis of trachea due to granulation
- Tracheo-oesophageal fistula
- Infection of tracheostomy site
- Tracheal irritation, ulceration and necrosis caused by overinflated cuff or excessive tube movement

Respiratory assessment

Patients present with a variety of conditions, and assessments need to be adapted to suit their needs. This section provides a basic framework for the subjective and objective respiratory assessment of a patient.

Database

- History of present condition
- Past medical history
- Drug history
- Family history
- Social history
  - support at home
  - home environment
  - occupation and hobbies
  - smoking

Subjective examination

- Patient's main concern
- Symptoms

- shortness of breath
- cough (productive or nonproductive)
- chest pain
- wheeze
- sputum and haemoptysis
- Other associated symptoms
  - fever
  - headache
  - fatigue
  - palpitations
  - nausea and vomiting
  - gastrointestinal reflux
  - urinary incontinence
- Functional ability/exercise tolerance

Objective examination

Charts

- Blood pressure
- Heart rate
- Temperature
- Oxygen requirement
- Oxygen saturation
- Respiratory rate
- Weight
- Peak flow
- Spirometry
- Fluid balance
- Urine output
- Medications

+ ITU/HDU charts

- Mode of ventilation
- FiO_2
- Heart rhythm
- Pressure support/volume control
- Airway pressure
- Tidal volume
- I:E ratio

- PEEP
- MAP
- CVP
- GCS
- ABGs
- Blood chemistry

X-rays and other diagnostic imaging (e.g. MRI, CT)

Observation

- General appearance
- Position
- Oxygen therapy
- Humidification
- Lines and drains
- Presence of wheeze or cough
- Sputum
  - colour
  - volume
  - viscosity
- Quality of voice
- Ability to talk in full sentences
- Skin colour
- Jugular venous pressure
- Oedema
- Clubbing
- Flapping tremor
- Chest
  - shape
  - breathing pattern
  - work of breathing
  - chest wall movement
  - respiratory rate

Palpation

- Chest excursion
- Chest wall tenderness or crepitus
- Skin hydration
- Trachea

- Percussion note
- Capillary refill

Auscultation

- Breath sounds
- Added sounds
- Voice sounds

Functional ability

Exercise tolerance

References and Further Reading

Coviello, J. (2016). *ECG interpretation made incredibly easy* (6th ed.). Philadelphia: Wolters Kluwer.

Crossman, A., & Neary, D. (2015). *Neuroanatomy: an illustrated colour text* (5 ed.). Elsevier.

Hampton, J. R. (2013). *ECG made easy* (8th ed.). Edinburgh: Churchill Livingstone.

Harden, B., Cross, J., Broad, M. A., Quint, N., Ritson, P., & Thomas, S. (2009). *Respiratory physiotherapy: an on-call survival guide* (2nd ed.). Edinburgh: Churchill Livingstone.

Hillegass, E. A. (2016). *Essentials of cardiopulmonary physical therapy* (4th ed.). St Louis: Elsevier.

Hough, A. (2018). *Hough's cardiorespiratory care: an evidence-based, problem-solving approach* (5th ed.). Edinburgh: Elsevier.

Main, E., & Denehy, L. (2016). *Cardiorespiratory physiotherapy: adults and paediatrics* (5th ed.). Elsevier.

Martini, F. H., Nath, J. L., & Batholomew, E. F. (2017). *Fundamentals of anatomy and physiology* (11th ed.). London: Pearson.

Thomas, A., Maxwell, L. J., Main, E., & Keilty, S. (2016). Clinical assessment. In E. Main & L. Denehy (Eds.), *Cardiorespiratory physiotherapy: adults and paediatrics* (5th ed., pp. 47–82). Elsevier.

Richards, A., & Edwards, S. (2012). *A nurse's survival guide to the ward* (3rd ed.). Edinburgh: Churchill Livingstone.

Ward, J., Ward, J., & Leach, R. M. (2015). *The respiratory system at a glance* (4th ed.). Chichester: John Wiley & Sons.

Whiteley, S. M., Bodenham, A., & Bellamy, M. C. (2010). *Churchill's pocketbook of intensive care* (3rd ed.). Edinburgh: Churchill Livingstone.

Heuer, A. J., & Scanlan, C. L. (2018). *Wilkins' clinical assessment in respiratory care* (8th ed.). St Louis: Elsevier.

SECTION

4

RESPIRATORY

Pathology

SECTION 5

Alphabetical listing of pathologies

Acute respiratory distress syndrome (ARDS)

ARDS can be caused by a wide variety of factors including pneumonia, sepsis, smoke inhalation, aspiration, major trauma and burns. As a result, the body launches an inflammatory response that affects the alveolar epithelium and pulmonary capillaries. In ARDS, the alveolar walls break down and the pulmonary capillaries become more permeable allowing plasma and blood to leak into the interstitial and alveolar spaces, while at the same time the capillaries become blocked with cellular debris and fibrin. The lungs become heavy, stiff and waterlogged, and the alveoli collapse. This leads to ventilation/perfusion mismatch and hypoxaemia, and patients normally require mechanical ventilatory support to achieve adequate gas exchange. Symptoms usually develop within 24–48 hours after the original injury or illness but can develop 5–10 days later.

AIDs (acquired immunodeficiency syndrome)

Caused by infection with the human immunodeficiency virus (HIV), which destroys a subgroup of lymphocytes and monocytes, resulting in suppression of the immune system. The virus enters the host cell and causes a mutation of its DNA so that the host cell becomes an infective agent (known as the provirus). Signs and symptoms include fever, malaise, painful throat, swollen lymph nodes and aching muscles in the initial period following infection. After a variable period of latency (1–15 years), weight loss, night sweats, long-lasting fever and diarrhoea occur as AIDS itself develops, which eventually progresses to the acquisition of major opportunistic infections and cancers such as pneumonia or Kaposi's sarcoma (a malignant skin tumour appearing as purple to dark brown plaques). Antiretroviral drugs are used to prolong the lives of infected individuals, although there is no cure or vaccine for the disease.

Alzheimer's disease

A form of dementia that is characterized by slow, progressive mental deterioration. Symptoms may start with mild forgetfulness, difficulty remembering names and faces or recent events and progress to memory failure, disorientation, speech disturbances, motor impairment and aggressive behaviour. It is the most common form of dementia and is distinguished by the presence of neuritic plaques (primarily in the hippocampus and parietal lobes), and neurofibrillary tangles (mainly affecting the pyramidal cells of the cortex).

Ankylosing spondylitis (axial spondyloarthritis)

A chronic inflammatory autoimmune disease involving the entheses (tendon, ligament and joint capsule insertions). The spine and sacroiliac joints are primarily involved, although other joints can be affected. The inflammatory process causes erosion of adjacent bone followed by ossification of the affected enthesis leading to progressively restricted joint movement. Over time, the spine and sacroiliac joints can become fused. Initial symptoms usually develop from the late teens to early 30s and include low back pain (with prolonged early morning stiffness that improves with movement), fatigue, buttock pain and nocturnal pain (with improvement on getting up). Males and females are equally affected. Can be associated with inflammation of the eye (uveitis/iritis), bowel (ulcerative colitis/Crohn's disease) and skin (psoriasis), as well as an increased risk of developing osteoporosis, vertebral fractures and cardiovascular disease. The cause is unknown.

Asthma

A chronic inflammatory disease of the airways that makes them hyperresponsive to a wide range of stimuli including allergens, pollution, infection, exercise and stress. As a result, the airways narrow, leading to coughing, wheezing, chest tightness and difficulty breathing. These symptoms can range from mild to severe and may even result in death.

Axonotmesis

A more serious peripheral nerve injury than neuropraxia, involving axonal and myelin degeneration distal to the injury (Wallerian degeneration) but with preservation of the Schwann cell basement membrane. Axonal regeneration is possible with nerve fibres regenerating at approximately 1 mm per day.

Baker's cyst

Distension of the popliteal bursa, which may be accompanied by herniation of the synovial membrane of the knee-joint capsule forming a fluid-filled sac at the back of the knee. Associated with rheumatoid arthritis and osteoarthritis.

Bell's palsy

An acute, lower motor neurone paralysis of the face, usually unilateral, related to inflammation and swelling of the facial nerve (VII) within the facial canal or at the stylomastoid foramen. Symptoms include inability to close the eye on the affected side, hyperacusis and impairment of taste. Good recovery is common.

Boutonnière deformity

A flexion deformity of the proximal interphalangeal joint combined with a hyperextension deformity of the distal interphalangeal joint. Caused by a rupture of the central slip of the extensor tendon at its insertion into the base of the middle phalanx. This causes the proximal phalanx to push upwards through the lateral slips. The most common causes are rheumatoid arthritis and direct trauma.

Broca's aphasia

See Expressive aphasia.

Bronchiectasis

Dilatation and destruction of the bronchi as a result of recurrent inflammation or infection. It may be present from birth (congenital bronchiectasis) or acquired as a result of another disorder (acquired bronchiectasis). Causes of infection include impaired mucociliary clearance due to congenital disorders such as primary ciliary dyskinesia or cystic fibrosis as well as bronchial obstruction and impaired inflammatory response, either acquired after a severe episode of inflammation or secondary to immunodeficiency. The inability of the airways to clear secretions in the bronchi leads to a vicious circle of infection, damage and obstruction of the bronchi. Clinical features include productive cough, episodic fever, pleuritic pain and night sweats. Patients may develop pneumothorax, respiratory and heart failure, emphysema and haemoptysis.

Bronchiolitis

A common respiratory problem affecting young infants. Caused by inflammation of the bronchioles due to infection by the human respiratory syncytial virus (RSV). Commonly occurs in winter. Signs and symptoms are similar to those of the common cold and include runny or blocked nose, temperature, difficulty feeding, a dry cough, dyspnoea and wheeze. In severe cases, hypoxia, cyanosis, tachypnoea and a refusal to eat may develop, and hospitalization is necessary.

Bronchitis

An inflammation of the bronchi. Acute bronchitis is commonly associated with viral respiratory infections, i.e. the common cold or influenza, causing a productive cough, fever and wheezing. Chronic bronchitis is defined as a cough productive of sputum for 3 months a year for more than 2 consecutive years. It is characterized by inflammation of the airways leading to permanent fibrotic changes, excessive mucus production and thickening of the bronchial wall. This results in sputum retention and narrowing and obstruction of the airways. In severe cases, irreversible narrowing of the airways leads to dyspnoea, cyanosis, hypoxia, hypercapnia and heart failure. These patients are often described as 'blue bloaters'.

Brown-Sequard syndrome

A neurological condition that occurs when there is damage to one-half of the spinal cord. Below the lesion, there is motor and proprioception loss on the same side and loss of pain and temperature on the opposite side.

Bulbar palsy

A bilateral or unilateral lower motor neurone lesion that affects the nerves supplying the bulbar muscles of the head and neck. Causes paralysis or weakness of the muscles of the jaw, face, palate, pharynx and larynx leading to impaired swallow, cough, gag reflex and speech.

Bursitis

Inflammation of the bursa caused by mechanical irritation or infection. Bursas that are commonly affected include the prepatellar, olecranon (can be associated with gout), subacromial, trochanteric, semimembranosus and the 'bunion' associated with hallux valgus. May or may not be painful.

Cauda equina syndrome

Caused by compression of the nerve roots in the lumbar spine leading to a characteristic set of features that include bilateral neurogenic sciatica, reduced perineal sensation, altered bladder function, loss of anal tone and sexual dysfunction. Patients presenting with symptoms of CES need immediate referral for investigation as early diagnosis is essential to prevent long-term bladder, bowel and sexual dysfunction, sensory and motor loss in lower limbs and possible paralysis.

Carpal tunnel syndrome

Compression of the median nerve as it passes beneath the flexor retinaculum. Often caused by inflammation due to rheumatoid arthritis, hypothyroidism, diabetes, trauma, repetitive movements, pregnancy or during menopause. Characterized by pain, numbness, tingling or burning sensation in the distribution of the median nerve (i.e. the radial three and a half fingers and nail beds and the associated area of the palm). Symptoms are often worse at night. Patients also complain of clumsiness performing fine movements of the hand, particularly on waking.

Cerebral palsy

An umbrella term for a variety of posture and movement disorders arising from permanent brain damage incurred before, during, or immediately after birth. The disorder is most frequently associated with premature births and is often complicated by other neurological problems including epilepsy, visual, hearing and sensory impairments, communication and feeding difficulties, cognitive and behavioural problems. Common causes include intrauterine infection, intrauterine cerebrovascular insult, birth asphyxia, postnatal meningitis and postnatal cerebrovascular insult. The most common disability is a spastic paralysis, which can be associated with choreoathetosis (irregular, repetitive, writhing and jerky movements).

Charcot-Marie-Tooth disease

A progressive hereditary disorder of the peripheral nerves that is characterized by gradual progressive distal weakness and wasting, mainly affecting the peroneal muscle in the leg. Early symptoms include difficulty running and foot deformities. The disease is slowly progressive, and in the late stages the arm muscles can also be involved. Also known as hereditary motor sensory neuropathy (HMSN).

Chondromalacia patellae

Refers to degeneration of the patella cartilage causing pain around or under the patella. Common among teenagers and young adults, especially girls, it is linked to structural changes and muscle imbalance associated with periods of rapid growth. This leads to excessive and uneven pressure on patella cartilage. May also result from an acute injury to the patella.

Chronic fatigue syndrome

See Myalgic encephalomyelitis.

Chronic obstructive pulmonary disease (COPD)

An umbrella term for respiratory disorders that lead to obstruction of the airways. COPD is associated mainly with emphysema and chronic bronchitis but also includes chronic asthma. Risk factors include smoking, recurrent infection, pollution and genetics. Symptoms include cough, dyspnoea, excessive mucus production and chest tightness. Patients may also develop oedema and heart failure.

Claw toe

A flexion deformity of both the proximal interphalangeal and the distal interphalangeal joints combined with an extension deformity of the metatarsophalangeal joint.

Coccydynia

Pain around the coccyx. Often due to trauma, such as a fall onto the buttocks, or childbirth; however, the cause is often unknown.

Compartment syndrome

Soft-tissue ischaemia caused by increased pressure in a fascial compartment of a limb. This increased pressure can have a number of causes, but the main ones are swelling following major trauma, a cast being applied too tightly over an injured limb, or repetitive strain injury. Signs and symptoms are pain, pale/plum colour, absent pulse, paraesthesia and loss of active movement. If left untreated, it leads to necrosis of nerve and muscle in the affected compartment, which is known as Volkmann's ischaemic contracture.

Complex regional pain syndrome (CRPS)

An umbrella term for a number of conditions, usually affecting the distal extremities, whose common features include unremitting severe pain (often described as burning) and autonomic changes in the affected region such as swelling, tenderness, restriction of movement, increased skin temperature, sweating, discoloration of the skin (usually blue or dusky red) and osteoporosis. CRPS is subdivided into two groups:

Group I – conditions in which minor or major trauma has occurred but there is no identifiable nerve injury, e.g. after Colles' fractures
Group II – conditions in which there has been an injury to a major peripheral nerve (e.g. sciatic nerve)

Contracted shoulder (Adhesive capsulitis)

A condition that affects the glenohumeral joint synovial capsule and is characterized by a significant restriction of active and passive shoulder movement.

The aetiology is unknown, but it has been linked to diabetes, heart disease, shoulder trauma or surgery, inflammatory disease, cervical disease and hyperthyroidism. The condition usually affects middle-aged individuals, particularly women. It normally follows three distinct phases, each lasting approximately 6–9 months (although this can be extremely variable):

Phase 1: increasing pain accompanied by increasing stiffness
Phase 2: decreasing pain with the stiffness remaining
Phase 3: decreasing stiffness and gradual return to normal function

Also known as frozen shoulder.

Coxa vara

Any condition that affects the angle between the femoral neck and shaft so that it is less than the normal 120–135°. It can either be congenital (present at birth), developmental (manifests clinically during early childhood and progresses with growth) or acquired (malunited and nonunited fractures, a slipped upper femoral epiphysis, Perthes' disease and bone 'softening', e.g. osteomalacia, Paget's disease).

Cubital tunnel syndrome

Compression of the ulnar nerve as it passes through the cubital tunnel (between the medial epicondyle and the olecranon). Symptoms include pain, weakness and dysaesthesia along the medial aspect of the elbow, forearm and hand.

Cystic fibrosis

A progressive genetic disorder of the mucus-secreting glands of the lungs, pancreas, gastrointestinal tract and sweat glands. Chloride ion secretion is reduced and sodium ion absorption is accelerated across the cell membrane resulting in the production of abnormally viscous mucus. This thickened mucus lines the intestine and lung leading to malabsorption, malnutrition and poor growth as well as recurrent respiratory infections that eventually lead to chronic lung disease. The increased concentration of sodium in sweat upsets the mineral balance in the blood and causes abnormal heart rhythms. Other complications include male infertility, diabetes mellitus, liver disease and vasculitis. The disease is eventually fatal.

De Quervain's syndrome

A painful condition affecting movement of the thumb that involves the extensor pollicis brevis and abductor pollicis longus tendons and sheaths within the first dorsal compartment of the wrist. Although the exact cause is not known, it is usually aggravated by activities involving repetitive movements of the hand or wrist.

Dermatomyositis

A rare autoimmune connective-tissue disease related to polymyositis that mainly affects adults between 40 and 60 years of age and children between 5 and 15 years of age. It is more common in women than men. Symptoms include weak, tired and inflamed muscles, swollen skin and a distinctive skin rash. In severe cases the heart and lungs can be affected.

Developmental coordination disorder

A neurodevelopmental condition affecting fine and/or gross motor coordination in children and adults. Early physical developmental milestones may be delayed (e.g. self-care, writing, riding a bike). However, a definitive diagnosis is not given before 5 years of age since developmental rates vary widely. Thought to be more common in boys and can be associated with nonmotor difficulties including problems with planning and organization as well as memory, perception, processing, articulation and speech. Often coexists with autism spectrum disorder, attention deficit hyperactivity disorder and learning and language disorders. Also known as dyspraxia.

Developmental dysplasia of the hip

Used to describe a spectrum of disorders causing hip dislocation either at birth or soon afterwards. The acetabulum is abnormally shallow so that the femoral head is easily displaced. Females and the left hip are more commonly affected.

Diabetes insipidus

A condition that leads to frequent excretion of large amounts of diluted urine. The symptoms of excessive thirst and urination are similar to diabetes mellitus, but the two conditions are unrelated. Urine excretion is governed by antidiuretic hormone (ADH), which is made in the hypothalamus and stored in the pituitary gland. Diabetes insipidus is caused by damage to the pituitary gland or by insensitivity of the kidneys to ADH. This leads to the body losing its ability to maintain fluid balance.

Diabetes mellitus

A chronic condition caused by the body's inability to produce or effectively use the hormone insulin to regulate the transfer of glucose from the blood into the cells. This leads to higher than normal levels of blood sugar. If not corrected, this can lead to coma, kidney failure and ultimately, death. In the long term, high levels of glucose can damage blood vessels, nerves and organs leading to cardiovascular disease, chronic renal failure, retinal damage and poor wound healing.

There are two types of diabetes:

Type I– little or no insulin is produced. Requires lifelong treatment with insulin injections, diet control and lifestyle adaptations.

Type II – the body produces inadequate amounts of insulin or is unable to utilize insulin effectively. Mainly occurs in people older than 40 years of age and is linked to obesity.

Diffuse idiopathic skeletal hyperostosis (DISH)

A condition that is characterized by widespread calcification and ossification of ligaments, tendons and joint capsule insertions. Mainly affects the spine with calcification of the anterior longitudinal ligament, which radiologically gives the appearance of candle wax dripping down the spine. Other joints may be affected with ossification of ligament and tendon insertions. Radiographically distinguishable from spondyloarthropathies and degenerative disc disease in that underlying bone and disc height are preserved and the facet joints are unaffected. It mainly affects men older than 50 years of age and in most cases it is asymptomatic, though some patients complain of stiffness and mild pain. The cause is unknown. Also known as Forestier's disease.

Duchenne muscular dystrophy

See Muscular dystrophy.

Dupuytren's contracture

Thickening and shortening of the palmar aponeurosis together with flexion contracture of one or more fingers. The cause is unknown.

Ehlers-Danlos Syndrome (EDS)

A group of heritable connective tissue disorders that arise from genetic alterations in collagen. It is characterized by joint hypermobility and often instability as well as fragility and hyperextensibility (stretchiness) of skin and other tissues of the body. There are 13 types of EDS, the most common being the hypermobile form (hEDS). Rarer types include classical EDS and vascular EDS. Clinical features of hEDS include painful and clicking joints, joint sprains, subluxations, dislocations, fatigue, cardiovascular symptoms, dysautonomia (tachycardia, hypotension, syncope), mechanical and neuropathic bowel dysfunction (hernia, reflux, sluggish bowel, constipation, chronic inflammation), prolapse (mitral, rectal, uterine), myopia, astigmatism, poor response to local anaesthetic, striae atrophicae and easily bruised skin. Classical EDS is associated with greater skin extensibility resulting in more obvious scarring and organ prolapse. Vascular EDS, considered to be the most serious form, is associated with a greater risk for rupture of the blood vessels, gut wall and uterus, which can be life threatening and life shortening.

Emphysema

The walls of the terminal bronchioles and alveoli are destroyed by inflammation and lose their elasticity. This causes excessive airway collapse on expiration, which traps air in the enlarged alveolar sacs. This irreversible airways obstruction leads to symptoms of dyspnoea, productive cough, wheeze, recurrent respiratory infection, hyperinflated chest and weight loss. These patients are often described as 'pink puffers' who may hyperventilate, typically overusing their accessory respiratory muscles, and breathe with pursed lips in order to maintain airway pressure to decrease the amount of airway collapse.

Empyema

A collection of pus in the pleural cavity following nearby lung infection. Can cause a buildup of pressure in the lung, which causes pain and shortness of breath.

Enteropathic arthritis

This form of chronic inflammatory arthritis is associated with ulcerative colitis or Crohn's disease, which are types of inflammatory bowel disease (IBD). It affects around one-fifth of IBD sufferers. Although it predominantly affects the peripheral joints such as the knees, ankles and elbows, it can also affect the spine.

Expressive aphasia (Broca's aphasia)

A lesion of Broca's area, on the inferior frontal cortex, causing nonfluent, hesitant speech that is characterized by poor grammar and reduced word output while meaning is preserved. Perseverance can occur and writing may be impaired, but comprehension remains relatively intact. Broca's area is near the motor cortex for the face and arm and so may be associated with weakness in these areas.

Fibromyalgia

A nonarticular rheumatological disorder associated with chronic, widespread pain lasting 3 months or more. It is associated with increased sensitivity to pain, fatigue, unrefreshing sleep and cognitive/memory problems. Other problems associated with fibromyalgia include depression, anxiety, morning stiffness and headaches. The cause and pathogenesis of fibromyalgia is unknown, but it can either develop on its own or together with other conditions such as rheumatoid arthritis or systemic lupus erythematosus.

Forestier's disease

See Diffuse idiopathic skeletal hyperostosis.

Freiberg's disease

Degenerative aseptic necrosis of the metatarsal head, usually the second metatarsal head, which mainly affects athletic girls 10–15 years of age.

Functional neurological disorder

Characterized by neurological symptoms such as weakness, tremor, movement disorders, sensory symptoms, dissociative (nonepileptic) attacks and blackouts, which are due to a problem with the functioning of the nervous system, rather than neurological disease. Previously known as conversion disorder.

Ganglion

An abnormal but harmless cystic swelling that often develops over a tendon sheath or joint capsule, especially on the back of the wrist.

Giant cell (temporal) arteritis

Characterized by inflammation of large- and medium-sized arteries, usually in the head and neck, resulting in a reduction in blood and oxygen supply to the target organ. It is sometimes called temporal arteritis because the arteries around the temples are usually affected. It only tends to develop in adults older than 50 years of age and is more common in women than in men. Giant cell arteritis is closely linked with polymyalgia rheumatica syndrome. Patients present with intractable throbbing headache, jaw claudication (pain when chewing or talking), vision loss and generalized muscle ache. Early diagnosis and treatment with steroids is essential to prevent visual loss or brainstem stroke, as well as to relieve the headache. The cause is unknown.

Golfer's elbow (medial epicondylitis)

Tendinopathy of the common origin of the forearm flexors causing pain and tenderness at the medial aspect of the elbow and down the forearm.

Gout

Characterized by attacks of acute joint inflammation secondary to hyperuricaemia (raised serum uric acid) where monosodium urate or uric acid crystals are deposited into the joint cavity. The disease usually affects middle-aged men and mainly affects the big toe. If the disease progresses, urates may be deposited in the kidney (stones) or the soft tissues (tophi), especially the ears. Further joint destruction can occur.

Guillain-Barré syndrome (GBS)

An acute inflammatory polyneuropathy that usually occurs 1–4 weeks after fever associated with viral infection or following immunization. Thought to be an autoimmune disorder, it leads to segmental demyelination of spinal roots and axons, denervation atrophy of muscle and inflammatory infiltration of the brain, liver, kidneys and lungs. Clinical features include loss of sensation in the hands and feet, symmetrical progressive ascending motor weakness, paralysis, muscle wasting, diminished reflexes, pain and autonomic disturbances. In severe cases, the respiratory and bulbar systems are affected and ventilation/tracheostomy may be required. Recovery is common.

Haemothorax

Blood in the pleural cavity. Commonly due to chest trauma but also found in patients with lung and pleural cancer and in those who have undergone thoracic or heart surgery.

Hallux valgus

A lateral deviation of the great toe at the metatarsophalangeal joint. The metatarsal head becomes prominent (bunion) and, along with the overlying bursa, may become inflamed.

Hammer toe

An extension deformity of the metatarsophalangeal joint, combined with a flexion deformity of the proximal interphalangeal joint. The second toe is the most commonly affected.

Herpes zoster

See Shingles.

Horner's syndrome

A group of symptoms caused by a lesion of the sympathetic pathways in the hypothalamus, brainstem, spinal cord, C8–T2 ventral spinal roots, superior cervical ganglion or internal carotid sheath. It causes ipsilateral pupil constriction, drooping of the upper eyelid and loss of facial sweating on the affected side of the face.

Huntingdon's disease

A hereditary disease caused by a defect in chromosome 4 that can be inherited from either parent. Onset is insidious and occurs between 35 and 50 years of age. Symptoms include sudden, involuntary movements (chorea) accompanied by behavioural changes and progressive dementia.

Hypermobility spectrum disorder (previously known as joint hypermobility syndrome)

Hypermobility describes a condition in which joint movement is in excess of normal range. In some cases this poses no problem to the individual, but in others it makes joints more susceptible to soft-tissue injury and internal derangement, arthritis, arthralgias and myalgias. Hypermobility spectrum disorder is used to describe those who are symptomatic due to their hypermobility but do not have a heritable disorder of connective tissue, such as EDS or Marfan syndrome. The clinical features and number of joints affected are highly variable and may include a history of dislocation, subluxation, sprains, tendonitis and proprioceptive deficit.

Hyperparathyroidism

Occurs when overactivity of the parathyroid glands leads to excessive secretion of parathyroid hormone (PTH), which regulates levels of calcium and phosphorus. Overproduction of PTH causes excessive extraction of calcium from the bones and leads to hypercalcaemia. Symptoms include fatigue, memory loss, renal stones and osteoporosis.

Hyperthyroidism

Occurs when the thyroid gland produces too much thyroxine, a hormone that regulates metabolism. This increase in metabolism causes most body functions to accelerate, and symptoms may include tachycardia, palpitations, hand tremors, nervousness, shortness of breath, irritability, anxiety, insomnia, fatigue, increased bowel movements, muscle weakness, heat intolerance, weight loss despite an increase in appetite, thinning of skin and fine brittle hair. Also known as overactive thyroid or thyrotoxicosis.

Hyperventilation syndrome

Breathing in excess of metabolic requirements, which causes low arterial carbon dioxide levels, leading to alkalosis and changes in potassium and calcium ion distribution. As a result, neuro-muscular excitability and vasoconstriction occur. Clinical features include lightheadedness, dizziness, chest pain, palpitations, breathlessness, tachycardia, anxiety, paraesthesia and tetanic cramps.

Hypothyroidism

Occurs when the thyroid gland does not produce enough thyroxine, a hormone that regulates metabolism. This decrease in metabolism causes most body functions to slow down, and symptoms may include tiredness, weight gain, dry skin and hair, cold intolerance, hoarse voice, memory loss, muscle cramps, constipation and depression. Also known as underactive thyroid.

Interstitial lung disease

An umbrella term for a wide range of respiratory disorders characterized by inflammation and, eventually, fibrosis of the lung connective tissue. The bronchioles, alveoli and vasculature may all be affected causing the lungs to stiffen and decrease in size. Examples of interstitial lung disease include fibrosing alveolitis, asbestosis, pneumoconiosis, bird fancier's or farmer's lung, systemic lupus erythematosus, scleroderma, rheumatoid disease, cryptogenic pulmonary fibrosis and sarcoidosis. Also known as diffuse parenchymal lung disease.

Jones fracture

A stress fracture of the proximal end of the fifth metatarsal.

Köhler's disease

A condition in which the navicular bone undergoes avascular necrosis. It usually affects children between 1 and 10 years of age (more commonly boys) with a peak between 3 and 7 years of age. The cause is unclear, but the disease usually resolves over time (1 month to 2 years) without any long-term consequences.

Locked-in syndrome

A rare neurological disorder characterized by total paralysis of all voluntary muscles except those controlling eye movement and some facial movements. It is caused by damage to the pons (brainstem). This may be due to traumatic brain injury, vascular disease, demyelinating diseases or overdose. Patients are unable to speak or move, but sight, hearing and cognition are normal. Prognosis for recovery is poor with most patients not regaining function.

Lung abscess

A pus-filled necrotic cavity within the lung parenchyma caused by infection.

Mallet finger

A flexion deformity of the distal interphalangeal joint due to damage to the extensor tendon at its insertion into the distal phalanx. The result is an inability to extend the distal phalanx.

March fracture

A stress fracture of the metatarsal. Usually affects the second or third metatarsal, but it can affect the fourth and fifth. Initially the fracture may not be visible on X-ray, but abundant callus is seen on later X-rays.

Marfan syndrome (MFS)

A heritable disorder of connective tissue that is thought to result from a mutation in the fibrillin gene. Patients present with a distinct collection of features known as the marfanoid habitus, which include a tall, slender body with long arms, hands, fingers, legs, feet and toes, flexible joints and scoliosis. Other features include pectus excavatum or carinatum, pes planus, mitral valve prolapse, and dislocation of the ocular lens. MFS also carries an increased risk for aortic aneurysm.

Meningitis

An acute inflammation of the meninges due to infection by bacteria or viruses. Age groups most at risk are those younger than 5, especially infants younger than 1, and adolescents between 15 and 19 years of age. The most common causes of bacterial meningitis in young children are *Neisseria meningitidis* (meningococcal meningitis) and *Haemophilus influenzae*. The classic triad of clinical features is fever, headache and neck stiffness. Skin rash and septic shock may occur where septicaemia has developed as a result of widespread meningococcal infection. Other signs in adults include confusion and photophobia. Onset of symptoms may be gradual or sudden; however, deterioration is rapid, often requiring intensive supportive therapy.

Meralgia paraesthetica

Pain, numbness and tingling in the anterolateral thigh caused by compression of the lateral cutaneous nerve as it passes under the inguinal ligament. Pregnancy, obesity and tight clothing are associated risk factors. Usually responds well to conservative treatment and resolves over time.

Morton's neuroma (metatarsalgia)

A fibrous thickening of the digital nerve as it travels between the metatarsals. Can be caused by irritation, trauma or compression. Usually occurs between the second and third metatarsal or the third and fourth metatarsal. Symptoms include burning, numbness, paraesthesia and pain in the ball of the foot. Also known as plantar neuroma and plantar digital neuritis.

Motor neurone disease

A group of progressive degenerative diseases of the motor system occurring in middle to late adult life, causing weakness, wasting and eventual paralysis of muscles. It primarily affects the anterior horn cells of the spinal cord, the motor nuclei of the brainstem and the corticospinal tracts. There are four main types:

Progressive muscle atrophy

Starts early in life, typically before 50 years of age. Affects the cervical region leading to atrophy of the muscles of the hand. Involvement spreads to the arms and shoulder girdle and may extend to the legs.

Amyotrophic lateral sclerosis

There are upper motor neurone changes as well as lower motor neurone changes. Characterized by weakness and atrophy in the hands, forearms and legs but may also spread to the body and face.

Progressive bulbar palsy

Caused by damage to the motor nuclei in the bulbar region in the brainstem, which results in wasting and paralysis of muscles of the mouth, jaw, larynx and pharynx. General features include pain and spasms, dyspnoea, dysphagia, dysarthria and sore eyes.

Primary lateral sclerosis

Occurs rarely. Causes weakness in the leg muscles, and some people may develop clumsiness in the hands or speech problems.

Multiple sclerosis

A chronic, progressive disease characterized by multiple demyelinating lesions (plaques) throughout the central nervous system. It predominantly affects young adults between 20 and 40 years of age and is more prevalent in women. The disease is usually characterized by recurrent relapses (attacks) followed by remissions, although some patients follow a chronic, progressive course. The plaques interfere with normal nerve impulses along the nerve fibre and the site of the lesions, and the degree of inflammation at each site leads to a variety of neurological signs and symptoms. Common symptoms include visual disturbances, ataxia, sensory and motor disturbances, bulbar dysfunction, fatigue, bladder and bowel symptoms, cognitive and emotional disturbances, pain and spasm.

There are four broad groups of MS:

Relapsing/remitting (RRMS)

Partial or complete recovery between relapses. The majority of people with MS (around 80%) are diagnosed with this form.

Secondary progressive (SPMS)

Slowly progressive deterioration with or without relapses. Those diagnosed with RRMS (about 50%) may go on to develop SPMS.

Benign (BMS)

One or two relapses with full recovery.

Primary progressive (PPMS)

Progression of neurological symptoms without relapses. Affects 10–15% of MS patients.

Muscular dystrophy

A group of genetically determined progressive muscle-wasting diseases. Duchenne muscular dystrophy is the most common and severe form among children, in which the affected muscle fibres degenerate and are replaced by fat and connective tissue. The condition affects boys between 3 and 5 years of age. Its clinical features include difficulty walking, pseudohypertrophy of proximal muscles, postural problems, diminished reflexes and difficulty standing from squatting (Gower's sign). Myotonic dystrophy is the most common form in adulthood, usually in the second decade. There are two types, with type 1 being more severe than type 2. Clinical features include myotonia (difficulty relaxing the muscles), ptosis and slow, progressive weakness of the face, neck and distal limb muscles. Cardiomyopathy with arrhythmias and gastrointestinal disturbances can occur.

Myalgic encephalomyelitis

A condition in which patients complain of long-term, persistent and debilitating fatigue along with other symptoms such as muscle pain, joint pain, disordered sleep, gastric disturbances, poor memory and concentration, headaches, sore throat and tender lymph nodes in the armpit and neck, though patients will not necessarily have all of them. Diagnosis is based on symptoms and tests that rule out other causes. No single cause of the disease has been established.

Myasthenia gravis

A disorder of the neuromuscular junction caused by an impaired ability of the neurotransmitter acetylcholine to induce muscular contraction, most likely due to an autoimmune destruction of the postsynaptic receptors for acetylcholine. It predominantly affects adolescents and young adults (mainly women) and is characterized by abnormal weakness and fatiguing of some or all muscle groups to the point of temporary paralysis. Onset of symptoms is usually gradual and includes drooping of the upper eyelid, double vision, dysarthria and weakness of other facial muscles.

Myeloma (also known as multiple myeloma)

A malignant condition in which abnormal plasma cells build up in the bone marrow. It can appear as both a tumour and/or an area of bone loss and tends to affect the spine (vertebral bodies), pelvis, ribs, skull, shoulder and hip girdles. It also interferes with the production of red blood cells and white blood cells and can lead to kidney damage. Because myeloma can occur at a number of sites in the bone marrow, it is often referred to as multiple myeloma. Symptoms include hypercalcaemia, anaemia, kidney damage, fatigue, infections, bone pain, fractures and weight loss. Older people (older than 50 years of age) are primarily affected.

Myositis ossificans

Growth of bone in the soft tissues near a joint that occurs after fracture or severe soft-tissue trauma, particularly around the elbow. Also occurs in a congenital progressive form, usually leading to early death during adolescence.

Myotonic dystrophy

See Muscular dystrophy.

Neuropraxia

The mildest type of peripheral nerve injury characterized by a transient and reversible loss of nerve conduction without structural damage to the axon. Causes include blunt trauma, traction-ischaemia from fracture-dislocation, compression-ischaemia (e.g.

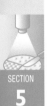

compartment syndrome), irradiation. Recovery occurs within 8–12 weeks.

Neurotmesis

The most serious peripheral nerve injury where the nerve and nerve sheath is disrupted. Surgical repair is necessary, though recovery is unpredictable.

Osgood-Schlatter's disease

Seen mainly in teenagers (boys slightly more than girls), it affects the tibial tubercle. Vigorous physical activity can cause the patellar tendon to pull at its attachment to the tibial tuberosity resulting in detachment of small cartilage fragments.

Osteoarthritis

A chronic disease of articular cartilage, associated with secondary changes in the underlying bone, causing joint inflammation and degeneration. Primarily affects the large, weight-bearing joints such as the knee and hip, resulting in pain, loss of movement and loss of normal function.

Osteochondritis

An umbrella term for a variety of conditions in which there is compression, fragmentation or separation of a piece of bone i.e. Osgood-Schlatter's disease, Osteochondritis dissecans, Perthes' disease, Scheuermann's disease, Sever's disease, Sinding-Larsen-Johansson's disease.

Osteochondritis dissecans

It occurs when a localized area of bone dies due to a lack of blood supply. Consequently, there is gradual localized separation of the cartilage and underlying bone. Can be caused by repetitive strain or trauma and mainly affects children and adolescents. The loose body can enter the joint space resulting in pain, swelling and reduced movement. The knee, elbow and ankle are the most commonly affected joints.

Osteogenesis imperfecta

A heritable disorder of connective tissue caused by an abnormal synthesis of type I collagen. As a result, bone is susceptible to fracture and deformity and connective tissue may also be affected. There are several different forms, which vary in appearance and severity. In its mildest form, features may include a history of fractures (which mainly occur before puberty), lax joints, low muscle tone, tinted sclera ranging from nearly white to dark blue or grey and adult-onset deafness. Those with a more severe form of the disease suffer short stature, progressive bone deformity and frequent fractures. Some types of the disease can be fatal in the perinatal period. Also known as brittle bone disease.

Osteomalacia

Softening of the bone caused by a deficiency in vitamin D from poor nutrition, lack of sunshine or problems absorbing or metabolizing vitamin D. A lack of vitamin D leads to incomplete calcification of the bones so that they become weak and easily fractured. This is particularly noticeable in the long bones, which become bowed. When this affects children, it is called rickets.

Osteomyelitis

An inflammation of the bone and bone marrow due to infection. The most common causes are infection of an open fracture or postoperatively after bone or joint surgery. The infection is often spread from another part of the body to the bone via the blood.

Osteoporosis

A reduction in bone density which results from the body being unable to form enough new bone or when too much calcium and phosphate is reabsorbed back into the body from existing bones. This leads to thin, weak, brittle bones that are susceptible to fracture. Osteoporosis is common in postmenopausal women, where a loss of ovarian function results in a reduction in oestrogen production. It can also be caused by prolonged disuse and non–weight bearing, endocrine disorders such as Cushing's disease, and steroid therapy.

Paget's disease

Characterized by an excessive amount of bone breakdown associated with abnormal bone formation causing the bones to become enlarged, deformed and weak. Normal architecture of the trabeculae is affected making the bones brittle. Paget's disease is usually confined to individual bones, although more than one bone can be affected. The pelvis, femur, and lower lumbar vertebrae are the most commonly affected. Also known as osteitis deformans. The cause remains unknown.

Parkinson's disease

A degenerative disease of the substantia nigra that reduces the amount of dopamine in the basal ganglia. Depletion of dopamine levels affects the ability of the basal ganglia to control movement, posture and coordination and leads to the characteristic symptoms of rigidity, slowness of voluntary movement, poor postural reflexes and resting tremor. Parkinson's has a gradual, insidious onset and affects mainly those between 50 and 65 years of age. Early symptoms of Parkinson's disease include aches and stiffness, difficulty with fine manipulative movements, slowness of walking, resting tremor of head, hands (pill rolling) and feet. Later symptoms may include shuffling gait, difficulties with speech, a masklike appearance and depression.

Pellegrini-Stieda syndrome

Local calcification of the femoral attachment of the medial collateral ligament (MCL), usually following direct trauma or a sprain/tear of the MCL. Signs and symptoms include chronic pain and tenderness, difficulty extending and twisting the knee, marked restriction of knee range of movement and a tender lump over the proximal portion of the knee.

Peripheral nerve injury

See Neuropraxia, Axonotmesis, Neurotmesis

Perthes' disease

A childhood condition which occurs when the blood flow to the upper femoral epiphysis is compromised, causing parts of the femoral head to become ischaemic and necrotic. The tissues of the femoral head become soft and fragmented but eventually reform over a period of several years as the blood vessels regrow. The reformed head is flatter and larger than the original, which can lead to deformity, shortening and secondary osteoarthritis. The cause is unknown.

Piriformis syndrome

Refers to irritation of the sciatic nerve by the piriformis muscle. Swelling of the muscle through injury or overuse is thought to compress on the sciatic nerve resulting in pain, numbness or tingling in the buttock that can extend along the posterior thigh and calf.

Plantar fasciitis

An inflammatory or degenerative condition affecting the plantar fascia. Pain is usually felt along the medial aspect of the calcaneal tuberosity where the plantar aponeurosis inserts and may extend down the proximal plantar fascia.

Pleural effusion

A collection of excess fluid in the pleural cavity which can be caused by a number of mechanisms:

- Increased hydrostatic pressure, e.g. congestive heart failure
- Decreased plasma-oncotic pressure, e.g. cirrhosis of the liver, malnutrition
- Increased capillary permeability, e.g. inflammation of the pleura
- Impaired lymphatic absorption, e.g. malignancy
- Communication with peritoneal space and fluid, e.g. ascites

The fluid can either be clear/straw-coloured and have a low protein content (known as a transudate), indicating a disturbance of the normal pressure in the lung, or it can be cloudy and have a high protein content (known as an exudate), indicating infection, inflammation or malignancy.

Pleurisy

Inflammation of the pleura causing severe pain as a result of friction between their adjoining surfaces. Pain is focused at the site of the inflammation and is increased with deep inspiration and coughing. Most commonly caused by a viral infection as well pneumonia, tuberculosis, rheumatic diseases and chest trauma.

Pneumonia

An inflammation of the lung tissue, mostly caused by bacterial or viral infection but also by fungi or aspiration of gastric contents. Pneumonia can be divided into two types:

- Community-acquired pneumonia: most commonly caused by the bacterium *Streptococcus pneumoniae*
- Hospital-acquired pneumonia: tends to be more serious as patients are often immunocompromised and they may be infected by bacteria resistant to antibiotics

The most common infective agents are bacteria such as *Pseudomonas*, *Klebsiella* and *Escherichia coli*. Clinical features include productive or dry cough, pleuritic pain, fever, fatigue and, after a few days, purulent and/or blood-stained sputum.

Pneumothorax

A collection of air in the pleural cavity following a lesion in the lung or trauma to the chest, which causes the lung to collapse. Clinical features include acute pain, dyspnoea and decreased movement of the chest wall on the affected side. Sometimes this can lead to significant impairment of respiration and/or circulation, known as a *tension pneumothorax*. This occurs when the amount of air pressure within the pleural cavity increases due to the formation of a one-way valve caused by damage to the visceral pleura, allowing air to enter on inspiration but preventing it from escaping on expiration. Clinical features include increased respiratory distress, cyanosis, hypotension, tachycardia and tracheal deviation. In severe cases, this can cause a mediastinal shift, which impairs venous return, leading to respiratory and cardiac arrest. Pneumothoraces are classified by how they are caused and divided into three types:

- Primary spontaneous pneumothorax: occurs without a known cause. Usually affects tall, thin young men, especially smokers

- Secondary spontaneous pneumothorax: occurs in the presence of underlying lung disease. Associated with diseases such as COPD, asthma, emphysema, cystic fibrosis and pneumonia
- Traumatic pneumothorax: caused by traumatic injury to the chest, e.g. perforation of lung tissue by fractured ribs or stab wound, or during medical procedures such as insertion of central venous lines, lung biopsies or mechanical ventilation

Poliomyelitis

Poliomyelitis is a highly contagious infectious disease caused by one of three types of poliovirus. The extent of the disease varies, with some people experiencing no or mild symptoms, while others develop the paralytic form of the disease. It can strike at any age, but affects mainly children younger than 5 years of age. The poliovirus destroys motor neurones in the anterior horn. The muscles of the legs are affected more often than those of the arm, but the paralysis can spread to the muscles of the thorax and abdomen. In the most severe form (bulbar polio), the motor neurones of the brainstem are attacked, reducing breathing capacity and causing difficulty in swallowing and speaking. Without respiratory support, bulbar polio can result in death.

Polyarteritis nodosa

A vasculitic syndrome where small- and medium-sized arteries are attacked by rogue immune cells causing inflammation and necrosis. Tissue supplied by the affected arteries, most commonly the skin, heart, kidneys and nervous system, is damaged by the impaired blood supply. Common manifestations are fever, renal failure, hypertension, neuritis, skin lesions, weight loss and muscle and joint pain.

Polymyalgia rheumatica

A vasculitic syndrome associated with fever and generalized pain and stiffness, especially in the shoulder and pelvic girdle areas. Other symptoms include overwhelming tiredness, loss of appetite, weight loss, anxiety and depression. Symptoms usually begin

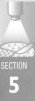

abruptly, and it mainly affects women older than 50 years of age.

Polymyositis

An autoimmune, inflammatory muscle disease of unknown aetiology causing progressive weakness of skeletal muscle. The muscles of the shoulder girdle, hip and pelvis are most commonly affected, although, less commonly, the distal musculature or swallowing can be affected. The muscles can ache and be tender to touch. The disease sometimes occurs with a skin rash over the upper body and is known as dermatomyositis.

Postpolio syndrome

A recurrence or progression of neuromuscular symptoms that appears in people who have recovered from acute paralytic poliomyelitis, usually 15–40 years after the original illness. Symptoms include progressive muscle weakness, severe fatigue and pain in the muscles and joints.

Postural (orthostatic) tachycardia syndrome (PoTS)

A form of cardiovascular autonomic dysfunction associated with excessive tachycardia on standing. It is defined as a heart rate increase of 30 beats per minute or more or a heart rate of more than 120 beats per minute within 10 minutes of standing, usually without an associated drop in blood pressure. It is often diagnosed with a Tilt Table Test. Symptoms can vary from mild to severe and included lightheadedness, fainting or almost fainting, headaches, fatigue, vision problems, palpitations, nausea, acrocyanosis (red/blue discoloration of the lower leg during standing caused by excessive venous pooling). It is most common in women between 13 and 50 years of age and is associated with several conditions including hypermobile Ehlers-Danlos syndrome, chronic fatigue syndrome, mast cell activation disorder, Sjögren's syndrome and antiphospholipid syndrome.

Primary ciliary dyskinesia

A genetic condition affecting the cilia causing abnormal ciliary activity and consequently, poor mucociliary clearance. Can be associated with situs inversus (the location of internal organs on the opposite side of the body), and when the two conditions exist together this is known as Kartagener's syndrome. Sperm can also be affected as they share a similar structure to cilia, leading to infertility in men. Clinical features include recurrent ear, sinus and chest infections, which can eventually lead to bronchiectasis.

Pseudobulbar palsy

An upper motor neurone lesion that affects the corticomotorneurone pathways and results in weakness and spasticity of the oral and pharyngeal musculature. Leads to slurring of speech and dysphagia. Patients also exhibit emotional incontinence. They are unable to control their emotional expression and may laugh or cry without apparent reason.

Psoriatic arthritis

A chronic inflammatory autoimmune disorder associated with psoriasis (a skin condition characterized by red, itchy, scaly patches) causing joints to become stiff, painful and swollen. Approximately 30% of people with psoriasis are affected, and it can either precede or follow the onset of the skin disease. Occasionally, psoriatic arthritis may occur in the absence of skin disease. Males and females are affected equally, and it is most common in middle age. Any joint can be involved, including the spine, though the most common pattern is for one large joint to be affected along with a number of small joints in the fingers or toes. Some people also develop psoriatic nail disease.

Pulmonary embolus

A blockage in the pulmonary artery most commonly caused by a blood clot that originates from one of the deep veins in the legs. This causes a ventilation/perfusion imbalance and leads to arterial hypoxaemia. Risk factors include prolonged bed rest or prolonged sitting (e.g. long flights), oral contraception, surgery, pregnancy, malignancy and fractures of the femur.

Pulmonary oedema

Accumulation of fluid in the lungs. Usually caused by left ventricular failure whereby a back pressure builds up in the

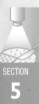

pulmonary veins, eventually causing fluid to be pushed from the veins into the alveoli. Pulmonary oedema can also be caused by myocardial infarction, damage to mitral or aortic valves, direct lung injury, severe infection, poisoning or fluid overload. Symptoms include shortness of breath, wheezing, sweating, tachycardia and coughing up white or pink-tinged frothy secretions.

Raynaud's phenomenon

A vasospastic disorder affecting the arterioles of the hands and feet, usually triggered by cold weather or emotional stress. The affected digits first turn pale and cold (ischaemia), then blue (cyanosis) and then bright red (reperfusion). The condition can either be primary, with no known cause, or secondary to an underlying disease such as systemic lupus erythematosus, polymyositis, rheumatoid arthritis and scleroderma.

Reactive arthritis

An inflammatory autoimmune disease that is caused by gastrointestinal or genitourinary infections. The syndrome is classically composed of joint pain, stiffness and swelling. It can be associated with urethritis and conjunctivitis. The disease usually resolves after 6 months, although in a small number of cases it can persist or recur. Also known as Reiter's syndrome.

Receptive aphasia (Wernicke's aphasia)

A lesion of Wernicke's area (posterolateral left temporal and inferior parietal language region of the left cortex) that results in an inability to process the meaning of spoken words and sentences. Writing and comprehension are greatly impaired, though the individual still has normal cognitive and intellectual abilities unrelated to speech or language. Speech is often fluent but nonsensical as the individual uses incorrect or made-up words. The patient is unaware of the language problem.

Right hemisphere language disorders

A term used to describe a range of communication problems associated with right hemisphere brain damage, i.e. CVA or traumatic brain injury, which are more subtle than those experienced by people with aphasia. Deficits include literal interpretations (inability to understand jokes, metaphors, irony, sarcasm, indirect requests and figurative language), difficulty in making inferences and identifying relevant information, inability to interpret body language and facial expressions, flat affect (monotonous speech pattern) and problems with conversational rules (i.e. turn-taking, verbosity).

Reiter's syndrome

See Reactive arthritis

Rheumatoid arthritis

A chronic, inflammatory autoimmune connective tissue disease involving the synovium. Can often affect several joints at the same time leading to destruction of the joint capsule, articular cartilage, bone, ligaments and tendons. Clinical features include joint deformity, stiffness, pain, swelling, heat, loss of movement and function. Other manifestations of the disease include subcutaneous nodules, muscle weakness, fatigue and anaemia. Can be associated with an increased risk for osteoporosis, vertebral fractures and cardiovascular disease. The disease is more common in young to middle-aged women, and the cause is unknown.

Rickets

See Osteomalacia

Sarcoidosis

An autoimmune disease that is characterized by the formation of nodules or lumps (granulomas) in one or more organs of the body. It mainly affects the lungs, eyes, skin, and lymph glands and may change how the organ functions. Patients commonly present with dyspnoea, persistent dry cough, skin rashes, or eye inflammation. They may also complain of being unwell or fatigued, and suffer fever and weight loss. In some cases, the patients are asymptomatic. The cause is unknown.

Scheuermann's disease

A condition caused by an abnormality in vertebral bone growth during adolescence resulting in the affected vertebrae becoming wedge-shaped, leading to an increased kyphosis of the spine. Degeneration of the intervertebral discs into the vertebral endplates can also occur. The thoracic spine is primarily affected, although it can sometimes affect the thoracolumbar and lumbar spine. The severity of the disease can vary. Some people experience little or no symptoms, while others experience severe pain, stiffness and loss of function. Boys are affected slightly more than girls. The cause is unknown.

Septic arthritis

An infection in the joint caused by bacteria (e.g. *Staphylococcus aureus*) or, rarely, by a virus or fungus. Patients present with pain, swelling, erythema, restricted movement and fever. In most cases, it only affects one joint. Risk factors include recent joint trauma, surgery or replacement, intravenous drug abuse, immunosuppressants, bacterial infection and existing joint conditions e.g. rheumatoid arthritis. Early diagnosis is essential, as delay can result in joint destruction. Also known as pyogenic arthritis and infective arthritis.

Sever's disease

A painful inflammation of the calcaneal apophysis that mainly affects growing, active children between 9 and 14 years of age. The pull of the Achilles tendon at its insertion causes traction of the apophysis, resulting in localized pain and tenderness of the heel. It is exacerbated by sports and activities like running and jumping.

Shingles

An infection of a sensory nerve and the area of skin that it supplies by the varicella/zoster virus (chickenpox). Following chickenpox infection, the virus remains dormant in a sensory nerve ganglion but can be reactivated later in life. Characterized by pain, paraesthesia and the appearance of a rash along the dermatomal distribution of the affected nerve. Mainly occurs in the trunk, although the face and other parts of the body can be affected. Occurs predominantly in the middle-aged and older population as well as the immunocompromised. Also known as herpes zoster.

Sickle-cell disease (Sickle-cell anaemia)

An inherited blood disorder characterized by atypical haemoglobin molecules that distort red blood cells into a rigid, sickle (crescent) shape. The affected blood cells break down prematurely leading to anaemia. Clinical features include shortness of breath, jaundice and delayed childhood growth. The cells can also stick to and obstruct smaller vessels causing tissue and organ ischaemia and subsequent damage. The lungs, kidneys, spleen and brain are particularly at risk and, as such, life-threatening complications such as stroke and pulmonary hypertension (leading sometimes to heart failure) can occur. Other complications include leg ulcers, retinopathy, avascular necrosis of the hip and other large joints, chronic pain and increased susceptibility to infection, particularly osteomyelitis. Although anyone can be a carrier of sickle cell disease, the trait is more common in people of African, Middle Eastern, Eastern Mediterranean and Indian origin.

Sinding-Larsen-Johansson's disease

Seen mainly in adolescents, it affects the inferior pole of the patella. Most commonly occurs in running and jumping sports, which cause the patella tendon to pull at its attachment at the inferior patellar pole. Results in fragmentation of the inferior patella and/or calcification in the proximal patellar tendon.

Sjögren's syndrome

An autoimmune connective tissue disorder in which the body's immune system attacks the moisture-producing glands, such as the salivary and tear glands. This produces the primary features of dry eyes and dry mouth. It can be primary or secondary to other autoimmune diseases such as rheumatoid arthritis, systemic sclerosis, systemic lupus erythematosus and polymyositis. Mainly affects women between 40 and 60 years of age.

Sleep apnoea

A cessation of breathing for more than 10 seconds caused by recurrent collapse of the upper airway leading to disturbed sleep. This may occur as a result of loss of muscle tone in the pharynx as the patient relaxes during sleep (obstructive sleep apnoea) and is usually associated with obesity or enlarged tonsils or adenoids. It may also be caused by abnormal central nervous system control of breathing (central sleep apnoea) or occur as a result of a restrictive disorder of the chest wall, e.g. scoliosis or ankylosing spondylitis, where normal use of accessory respiratory muscles is inhibited during sleep. Pulmonary hypertension, respiratory and/or heart failure may develop in severe cases.

Spina bifida

A developmental defect that occurs in early pregnancy in which there is incomplete closure of the neural tube. The posterior part of the affected vertebrae does not fuse, leaving a gap or split. There are three main types:

Spina bifida occulta

Mild form in which there is no damage to the meninges or spinal cord. The defect is covered with skin that may be dimpled, pigmented or hairy. In the vast majority of cases, it presents with no symptoms. However, in some cases the spinal cord may become tethered against the vertebrae, with possible impairment of mobility or bladder control.

Spina bifida cystica

When a blisterlike sac or cyst balloons out through the opening in the vertebrae. There are two forms:

Meningocele: the spinal cord and nerves remain in the spinal canal, but the meninges and cerebrospinal fluid balloon out through the opening in the vertebrae, forming a sac. This is the least common form of spina bifida.

Myelomeningocele: the spinal cord and nerves are pushed out through the opening, along with the meninges and cerebrospinal fluid. The spinal cord at this level is damaged leading to paralysis and loss of sensation below the affected segment. This is the most serious and more common form and is often associated with hydrocephalus.

Spinal muscular atrophies (SMA)

A group of inherited degenerative disorders of the anterior horn cell causing muscle atrophy. There are three main types, which are classified by age of onset:

SMA I (Werdnig–Hoffman disease) is the most severe form, with onset from preterm to 6 months of age. It causes weakness and hypotonia ('floppy' babies) leading to death within 3 years.

SMA II (intermediate type) usually develops between 6 and 15 months of age. It has the same pathological features as SMA I but progresses more slowly.

SMA III (Wohlfart-Kugelberg-Welander disease) has a late onset, between 1 year of age and adolescence, leading to progressive, proximal limb weakness.

SMA IV (*adult-onset SMA*) develops in early adulthood. It is a milder form of the condition and causes mild to moderate muscle weakness.

Spinal stenosis

Narrowing of the spinal canal, nerve root canals or intervertebral foramina. May be caused by a number of factors, including loss of disc height, osteophytes, facet hypertrophy, disc prolapse and hypertrophic ligamentum flavum.

Compression of the nerve root may lead to radiating leg or arm pain, numbness and paraesthesia in the affected dermatome, muscle weakness, neurogenic claudication and low back pain. In severe cases, the spinal cord may be compromised.

Spondyloarthritis (also known as seronegative spondyloarthropathy)

A group of inflammatory joint disorders that include ankylosing spondylitis, psoriatic arthritis, reactive arthritis, enteropathic arthritis, undifferentiated spondyloarthritis. They all share notable characteristics: the spine is usually affected, though other large joints are occasionally implicated; there is a strong link to human leukocyte antigen HLA-B27; there is an absence of rheumatoid factor in the blood; enthesopathy (inflammation of the ligaments and tendon where they attach to bone) commonly occurs, and onset is usually before 40 years of age.

Spondylolisthesis

A spontaneous forward displacement of one vertebral body upon the segment below it (usually L5/S1). Displacement may be severe, causing compression of the cauda equina, requiring urgent surgical intervention. Spondylolisthesis is classified according to its cause:

I Dysplastic – congenital
II Isthmic – fatigue fracture of the pars interarticularis due to overuse
III Degenerative – osteoarthritis
IV Traumatic – acute fracture
V Pathological – weakening of the pars interarticularis by a tumour, osteoporosis, tuberculosis or Paget's disease

In rare cases, the displacement may be backwards, known as a retrolisthesis.

Spondylolysis

A defect in the pars interarticularis of the lumbar vertebrae (usually L5), often the result of a fatigue fracture. It can be unilateral or bilateral and may or may not progress to spondylolisthesis.

Spondylosis

Degeneration and narrowing of the intervertebral discs leading to the formation of osteophytes at the joint margin and arthritic changes of the facet joints. The lowest three cervical joints are most commonly affected causing neck pain and stiffness, sometimes with radiation to the upper limbs, although the condition may remain symptomless. Can also occur in the lumbar and thoracic spine. In some cases, osteophytes may encroach sufficiently upon an intervertebral foramen to cause nerve root pressure signs, or, more rarely, the spinal canal to cause dysfunction in all four limbs and possibly the bladder. The vertebral artery can also be involved.

Stroke/cerebrovascular accident (CVA)

A condition in which part of the brain is suddenly severely damaged or destroyed as a consequence of an interruption to the flow of blood in the brain. This interruption may be caused by a blood clot (ischaemic stroke) or by a ruptured blood vessel (haemorrhagic stroke), either within the brain (intracerebral) or around the brain (subarachnoid). The most common symptoms of stroke are numbness, weakness or paralysis on one side of the body, contralateral to the side of the brain in which the cerebrovascular accident occurred. Other symptoms include dysphasia, dysphagia, dysarthria, dyspraxia, disturbance of vision and perception, inattention or unilateral neglect, and memory or attention problems. When symptoms resolve within 24 hours, this is known as a transient ischaemic attack (TIA).

Swan neck deformity

A hyperextension deformity of the proximal interphalangeal joint combined with a flexion deformity of the distal interphalangeal joints and, sometimes, a flexion deformity of the metacarpophalangeal joints due to failure of the proximal interphalangeal joint's volar/palmar plate. Usually seen in rheumatoid arthritis, but can be a result of injury.

Syringomyelia

A rare disorder in which a longitudinal cavity (syrinx) forms within the central spinal cord. The condition can be congenital or acquired following trauma (e.g. hyperextension injuries of the neck) or secondary to a space-occupying lesion. The lower cervical segments are usually affected, though the cavity can extend into the brainstem (syringobulbia). Symptoms vary according to the location and extent of the cavity but include dissociated sensory loss (loss of temperature and pain with intact proprioception) often occurring in a "capelike" distribution over the back, arms and hands. Paralysis and weakness can also occur.

Systemic lupus erythematosus (SLE)

A chronic, inflammatory autoimmune connective tissue disorder involving the skin, joints and internal organs. Clinical features and severity can vary widely depending on the area affected but may include butterfly rash on face, polyarthritis, vasculitis, Raynaud's disease, anaemia, hypertension, neurological disorders, renal disease, pleurisy and alopecia. Of those affected by the disease, around 90% are women.

Systemic sclerosis (scleroderma)

An autoimmune connective tissue disorder that causes an increase in collagen metabolism. Excessive collagen deposits cause damage to microscopic blood vessels in the skin (scleroderma) and other organs (systemic sclerosis), leading to fibrosis and degeneration. Any organ can be affected, and its effects can be localized or diffuse, as well as progressive. Middle-aged women are most commonly affected. Clinical features include oedema of hands and feet, contractures and finger deformities, alteration of facial features and dry, shiny, tight skin.

Talipes equinovarus

A common deformity of the foot and ankle, often congenital, where the foot is plantarflexed, adducted and supinated. This deformity can either be fixed (structural talipes) or passively corrected (positional talipes). Males are more commonly affected. Also known as clubfoot.

Talipes calcaneovalgus

A deformity of the foot and ankle, usually postural, where the foot is dorsiflexed and everted, and is resistant to plantarflexion. Common in breech births, and usually resolves within 12 weeks. Can be associated with hip dysplasia and leg length discrepancy.

Tarsal tunnel syndrome

Compression of the posterior tibial nerve or its branches as it passes through the tarsal tunnel (behind the medial malleolus). Symptoms include pain, dysaesthesia and weakness in the medial and plantar aspects of the foot and ankle. Can be confused with plantar fasciitis.

Tennis elbow (lateral epicondylitis)

Tendinopathy of the common origin of the forearm extensors causing pain and tenderness at the lateral aspect of the elbow and down the forearm.

Tenosynovitis

Inflammation of the synovial lining of a tendon sheath caused by mechanical irritation or infection, often associated with overuse and repetitive movements.

Thoracic outlet syndrome

An umbrella term for a group of conditions that result from compression of the neurovascular bundle in the cervicoaxillary canal. Common sites of compression are the costoclavicular space (between the first rib and the clavicle) and the triangle between the anterior scalene, middle scalene and first rib. Causes include muscle shortening and spasm, poor posture, stretching of the lower trunk of the brachial plexus, traumatic structural changes, or, more rarely, congenital anatomical abnormalities such as an enlarged C7 transverse process, cervical rib or clavicular bony abnormality. Clinical features include paraesthesia, pain, subjective weakness, oedema, pallor, discoloration or venous engorgement involving the neck and affected shoulder and upper limb.

Torticollis

Refers to the position of the neck in a number of conditions (rotated and tilted to one side). From the Latin *torti* meaning twisted and *collis* meaning neck.

Congenital torticollis

Caused by injury, and possible contracture, of the sternocleidomastoid by birth trauma or malpositioning in the womb. Seen in babies and young children.

Acquired torticollis

Acute torticollis (wry neck) is caused by spasm of the neck muscles (usually trapezius and sternocleidomastoid) that often results from a poor sleeping position. Usually resolves within a few days. *Spasmodic torticollis* is a focal dystonia caused by disease of the central nervous system which leads to prolonged and involuntary muscle contraction.

Transverse myelitis

A demyelinating disorder of the spinal cord in which inflammation spreads more or less completely across the tissue of the spinal cord resulting in a loss of its normal function to transmit nerve impulses. Paralysis and numbness affect the legs and trunk below the level of diseased tissue. Causes include immune system disorders, infection (viral, bacterial, fungal) and vascular disorders. Some patients progress to multiple sclerosis. Recovery varies.

Trigeminal neuralgia

A condition that is characterized by brief attacks of severe, sharp, stabbing facial pain in the territory of one or more divisions of the trigeminal nerve (cranial nerve V). It can be caused by degeneration or compression of the nerve, though the cause is often unknown. Attacks can last for several days or weeks, after which the patient may be pain-free for months.

Trigger finger

A condition that is characterized by catching, "popping" or locking of one of the fingers when it is flexed or extended. This is caused by inflammation and hypertrophy of the flexor tendon sheath that restricts the motion of the flexor tendon. The ring finger is the most commonly affected digit. It is more common in people with Type 1 diabetes and is also associated with rheumatoid arthritis and amyloidosis.

Tuberculosis

An infection caused by the bacterium *Mycobacterium tuberculosis*. It is spread when an individual with the disease coughs or sneezes, releasing the bacteria into the air, where it can be inhaled by someone else. In most healthy people, the body's natural defense kills the bacteria and no symptoms develop. In other cases, the body is unable to kill the bacteria, but it can prevent it spreading. Although the bacteria remains in the body, there are no symptoms and the person is not infectious to others. This is termed *latent TB*.

If the body fails to kill the bacteria or prevent it spreading it is termed *active TB*. Any tissue can be infected, but the lungs are the most common site. Other sites of infection include lymph nodes, bones, gastrointestinal tract, kidneys, skin and meninges. Latent TB can develop into active TB if the body's immune system becomes weakened following infection, inadequate immunity and malnutrition. Clinical features include persistent cough, haemoptysis, weight loss, fatigue, fever and night sweats.

Wernicke's aphasia

See Receptive aphasia

Diagnostic imaging

Plain radiography (X-rays)

An image formed by exposure to short wavelengths of electromagnetic radiation (X-rays) that pass through the body and hit a photographic receptor (radiographic plate or film) placed behind the patient's body. The X-rays pass through soft tissue, such as muscle, skin and organs, and turn the plate black, whereas hard tissue, such as bone, blocks the X-rays leaving the film white. Useful for detecting fractures, dislocations and many bony abnormalities including degenerative joint disease, spondylolisthesis, infections, tumours, avascular necrosis and metabolic bone diseases. Two views in planes at right angles to each other, usually anteroposterior and lateral, are usually required in order to adequately examine a region.

Can be used in conjunction with the instillation of iodinated contrast material into various structures of the body. These block the X-rays and help visualize the structure:

Angiography (blood vessels): cerebral aneurysms, vascular malformations and occluded or stenosed arteries and veins

Arthrography (joints): internal derangements of joints

Discography (intervertebral disc space): disc pathology

Myelography (thecal sac): compressive lesions of the spinal cord and cauda equina

Tenography (tendon sheath): tendon pathology and ligament ruptures

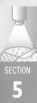

Computed tomography (CT)

Involves scanning part of the body from several angles by rotating a thin X-ray beam and detector around it. The data from the X-rays are then compared and reconstructed by computer to produce a cross-sectional image, which can be manipulated to emphasize bony or soft-tissue structures. Provides good detail of bony structures, especially cortical bone, and is particularly useful for complex fractures and dislocations as well as for osteochondral lesions, stress fractures, loose bodies and certain spinal pathologies such as stenosis and disc herniation. It can also be used for diagnosing aneurysms, brain tumours and brain damage and detecting tumours and abscesses throughout the body. As with plain film radiography, it can also be used in conjunction with the administration of iodinated contrast material into various body structures to image the brain, neck, chest, abdomen and pelvis.

Magnetic resonance imaging (MRI)

A cross-sectional image is formed by placing the body in a powerful magnetic field and using radiofrequency pulses to excite hydrogen nuclei within tissue cells. The signals emitted by the nuclei are measured and reconstructed by computer to create an image of soft tissue and bone. Different pulse sequences are used to accentuate different characteristics of tissue. T1-weighted images show good anatomical detail with fluid being dark and fat being bright. T2-weighted images are better at identifying soft tissue pathology, but anatomical detail is less clear. Fluid appears bright.

MRI provides superior soft-tissue contrast in multiple imaging planes and is used to examine the central nervous, musculoskeletal and cardiovascular systems. MRI has no known adverse physiological effects. It is often used with gadolinium, an intravenous contrast agent, to improve diagnostic accuracy (T1-weighted). Patients with a cardiac pacemaker, brain aneurysm clip or other metallic implants with the exception of those attached to bone, i.e. prosthetic joints, cannot undergo MRI.

Radionuclide scanning

Involves the administration of a radioactive label (radioisotope) along with a biologically active substance that is readily taken up by the tissue being examined, e.g. iodine for the thyroid gland. The radioisotope emits a particular type of radiation that can be picked up by gamma ray cameras or detectors as it travels through the body. Highly active cells in the target organ will take up more of the radionuclide and emit more gamma rays resulting in 'hot spots'. It is used to identify areas of abnormal pathology. Bone scans detect areas of increased activity and can pick up metastatic disease, infection (osteomyelitis) and fractures. It can also be used to investigate kidney, liver and spleen function, coronary blood flow and thyroid activity and to detect pulmonary emboli in the lungs.

Dual-energy X-ray absorptiometry (DEXA) scanning

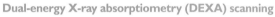

The most commonly used technique to measure bone mineral density. Two low-dose photon (X-ray) beams of different energies are transmitted through the bone being examined and are measured by a detector on the other side of the patient. The denser the bone, the fewer the X-rays that reach the detector. Used to diagnose and grade osteoporosis and assess the risk of a particular bone becoming fractured. The World Health Organization has defined bone mass according to the DEXA scan's T-scores, which are standard deviation (SD) measurements referenced to the young adult mean.

Normal: not more than 1 standard deviation below the average value

Osteopenia: more than 1 but less than 2.5 standard deviations below the average value

Osteoporosis: more than 2.5 standard deviations below the average value

Ultrasound

Involves high-frequency sound waves being directed into the body via a transducer, which are then reflected back from different tissue interfaces and converted into a real-time image. Can be used to examine a broad range of soft-tissue structures, such as the abdomen, peripheral musculoskeletal system, fetus in pregnancy, thyroid gland, eyes, neck, prostate and blood flow (Doppler). However, it cannot penetrate bone or deep structures.

Electrodiagnostic tests

Electroencephalography (EEG)

A technique that records the electrical activity of the brain via electrodes attached to the scalp. Used in the diagnosis of epilepsy, coma and certain forms of encephalitis.

Evoked potentials (EP)

A technique that studies nerve conduction of specific sensory pathways within the brain by measuring the time taken for the brain to respond to a stimulus. The stimulus may either be visual (e.g. flashed light, which measures conduction in the occipital pathways), auditory (e.g. click, which measures conduction in the auditory pathways) or somatosensory (e.g. electrical stimulation of a peripheral nerve, which measures conduction in the parietal cortex). Used for detecting multiple sclerosis, brainstem and cerebellopontine angle lesions (e.g. acoustic neuroma), various cerebral metabolic disorders in infants and children as well as lesions in the sensory pathways (e.g. brachial plexus injury and spinal cord tumour).

Nerve conduction studies

Measures conduction along a sensory or motor peripheral nerve following stimulation of that nerve from two different sites. The conduction velocity is calculated by dividing the distance between the two sites by the difference in conduction times between the two sites. Useful in the diagnosis of nerve entrapments (e.g. carpal tunnel syndrome), peripheral neuropathies, motor and sensory nerve damage and multifocal motor neuropathy.

Electromyography (EMG)

Involves the insertion of a needle electrode into muscle to record spontaneous and induced electrical activity within that particular muscle. Used in the diagnosis of a broad range of myopathies and neuropathies.

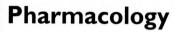

Pharmacology

Drug classes

ACE inhibitors

Angiotensin-converting enzyme (ACE) inhibitors allow blood vessels to dilate by preventing the formation of angiotensin II, a powerful artery constrictor. Used in the treatment of heart failure, hypertension, diabetic nephropathy and post–myocardial infarction.

Antibiotics

Used to treat bacterial disorders ranging from minor infections to deadly diseases. Antibiotics work by destroying the bacteria or preventing them from multiplying while the body's immune system works to clear the invading organism. There are different classes of antibiotic, which include penicillins (amoxicillin, ampicillin, benzylpenicillin, flucloxacillin), cephalosporins (cefaclor, cefotaxime, cefuroxime), macrolides (clarithromycin, erythromycin), tetracyclines (tetracycline), aminoglycosides (gentamicin) and glycopeptides (vancomycin).

Antiemetics

Act by blocking signals to the vomiting centre in the brain, which triggers the vomiting reflex. Used to prevent or treat vomiting and nausea caused by motion sickness, vertigo and digestive tract infection and to counteract the common side effects of some drugs.

Antiepileptics

Used to prevent or terminate epileptic seizures. There are several types of epilepsy, each treated by a specific antiepileptic medication. It is therefore essential to classify the type of seizure in order to treat it effectively and minimize common side effects.

Antiretrovirals

Used to treat the human immunodeficiency virus (HIV). Standard antiretroviral therapy uses a combination of antiretroviral drugs to suppress the HIV virus, slow down the progression of the disease and prevent its transmission.

Antiretrovirals work in a number of different ways:

Reverse transcriptase inhibitors – reduce the activity of the reverse transcriptase enzyme, which is vital for virus replication. They are divided according to their chemical structure into nucleoside reverse-transcriptase inhibitors (NRTIs), nucleotide reverse-transcriptase inhibitors (NtRTIs) and non-nucleoside reverse-transcriptase inhibitors (NNRTIs).

Protease inhibitors – interfere with the protease enzyme and interfere with virus replication.

Entry inhibitors – prevent the HIV virus from entering human cells. They are divided according to their mechanism of action into *entry blockers* and *fusion inhibitors*.

Integrase inhibitors – target the integrase enzyme, which is essential for integrating viral DNA into the human cell.

To reduce the development of drug resistance, the drugs are used in combination, known as HAART (highly active antiretroviral therapy). Current treatment aims to act at different phases of the viral life cycle and is usually initiated with a combination of two NRTIs plus an NNRTI or a protease inhibitor. Antiretrovirals are not a cure for HIV, but they increase life expectancy considerably. However, they are toxic, and treatment regimens must be carefully balanced.

β-blockers

Prevent stimulation of the β-adrenoreceptors in the heart muscle (mainly β_1-receptors) and peripheral vasculature, bronchi, pancreas and liver (mainly β_2-receptors). Used to treat hypertension, angina, myocardial infarction, arrhythmias and thyrotoxicosis. Can also be used to alleviate some symptoms of anxiety. Since blocking β-adrenoreceptors in the lungs can lead to constriction of air passages, care needs to be taken when treating patients with asthma or COPD.

Benzodiazepines

Increase the inhibitory effect of GABA, which depresses brain cell activity in the higher centres of the brain controlling

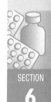

consciousness. Used for anxiety, insomnia, convulsions, sedation for medical procedures and alcohol withdrawal.

Bronchodilators

Dilate the airways to assist breathing when constricted or congested with mucus. There are two main types:

Sympathomimetics (i.e. salbutamol) stimulate β_2-adrenoreceptors on the surface of bronchial smooth muscle cells causing the muscle to relax.

Anticholinergics (i.e. ipratropium bromide) act by blocking the neurotransmitters that trigger muscle contraction.

Both are used to treat asthma and other conditions associated with reversible airways obstruction such as COPD.

Calcium channel blockers

Interfere with the transport of calcium ions through the cell walls of cardiac and vascular smooth muscle. Reduce the contractility of the heart, depress the formation and conduction of impulses in the heart and cause peripheral vasodilation. Used to treat angina, hypertension and arrhythmias.

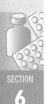

Corticosteroids

Natural or synthetic hormones that act on metabolism and tissue inflammation. They reduce inflammation by inhibiting the formation of inflammatory mediators, e.g. prostaglandins. Used to control many inflammatory disorders thought to be caused by excessive or inappropriate activity of the immune system, e.g. asthma, inflammatory bowel disease, rheumatoid arthritis, lupus, eczema, as well as inflammation caused by strain and damage to muscles and tendons.

The term *corticosteroids* refers to glucocorticoids and mineralocorticoids, but they each have different effects. Glucocorticoids' primary role is to reduce inflammation, while mineralocorticoids regulate the electrolyte and fluid balance of the body.

Diuretics

Work on the kidneys to increase the amount of sodium and water excreted. There are different types of diuretic that work on the nephron:

Thiazides (bendroflumethiazide/bendrofluazide)
Loop (furosemide/frusemide, bumetanide)
Potassium-sparing (amiloride, spironolactone)
Osmotic (mannitol)
Carbonic anhydrase inhibitors (acetazolamide, dorzolamide)

Used to treat hypertension (thiazides), chronic heart failure and oedema (loop diuretics, thiazides or a combination of both), glaucoma (carbonic anhydrase inhibitors or osmotic), raised intracranial pressure (osmotic).

Disease-modifying antirheumatic drugs (DMARDs)

A group of medicines commonly used to treat types of inflammatory disease such as rheumatoid arthritis, ankylosing spondylitis, psoriatic arthritis, inflammatory bowel disease, plaque psoriasis, systemic lupus erythematosus and juvenile idiopathic arthritis. They work via different mechanisms to suppress disease activity and reduce associated joint damage.

They can be broadly split into two categories:

Conventional DMARDs – refers to the traditional, nonbiological drugs, such as methotrexate, sulfasalazine and hydroxychloroquine.
Biological DMARDS – target particular molecules involved in the pathological immune response such as tumour necrosis factor alpha (TNFα). Examples include etanercept and adalimumab.

Inotropes

Work by increasing the contractility of the heart muscle. They can be divided into three groups:

Cardiac glycosides (i.e. digoxin) assist activity of the heart muscle by increasing intracellular calcium storage in myocardial cells. Used for heart failure and supraventricular arrhythmias.

Sympathomimetics (i.e. dobutamine, dopamine) stimulate β_1-receptors on the heart, which increase the rate and force of myocardial contraction. Provide inotropic support in infarction, cardiac surgery, cardiomyopathies, septic shock and cardiogenic shock.

Phosphodiesterase inhibitors (i.e. milrinone) inactivate cyclic AMP, which increases the force of myocardial contraction and relaxes vascular smooth muscle. Used to treat congestive heart failure.

Mucolytics

Reduce the viscosity of bronchopulmonary secretions by breaking down their molecular complexes. Used to treat excessive or thickened mucus secretions.

Nonsteroidal anti-inflammatory drugs (NSAIDs)

Inhibit the production of prostaglandins, which are responsible for inflammation and pain following tissue damage. They are called nonsteroidals to distinguish them from corticosteroids, which have a similar function. Used for inflammatory diseases, pain and pyrexia.

Opioids

Have a strong analgesic effect and are used to treat moderate to severe pain arising from surgery, cancer, acute trauma and terminal illness. Opioids reduce pain by binding to opioid receptors, which decreases nerve excitability, thereby reducing the transmission of nociceptive impulses to the brain. Opioid receptors are mainly found in the spinal cord, brain, peripheral sensory neurons and in the gastrointestinal tract. As well as their analgesic effects, opioids can produce a state of relaxation and euphoria, which can lead to abuse and addiction. Side effects include nausea and vomiting, constipation, respiratory depression and drowsiness.

A–Z of drugs

Abacavir (antiretroviral – NRTI)

Used in combination with other antiretroviral drugs to treat HIV infection.

Common side effects: nausea, vomiting, loss of appetite, diarrhea, headaches, fatigue, hypersensitivity reactions.

Acetylcysteine (mucolytic)

Reduces the viscosity of secretions associated with impaired or abnormal mucus production. Also used as an antidote for paracetamol overdose.
Common side effects: hypersensitivity-like reactions, rashes, nausea, vomiting, anaphylaxis (in children).

Aciclovir (antiviral)

Used against infections caused by herpes virus (herpes simplex and varicella-zoster).
Common side effects: rare.

Adalimumab (biological DMARD)

Used to treat moderate to severe rheumatoid arthritis, ankylosing spondylitis, psoriatic arthritis, Crohn's disease, ulcerative colitis, uveitis and juvenile idiopathic arthritis. Given by subcutaneous injection at two-weekly intervals.
Common side effects: headache, skin rash, antibody development, injection site reaction (erythema, itching, pain, swelling), upper respiratory tract infection.

Adenosine (antiarrhythmic)

Reverses supraventricular tachycardias to sinus rhythm.
Common side effects: facial flushing, dyspnoea, headache, nausea, lightheadedness, chest pain.

Adrenaline/epinephrine (sympathomimetic agent)

Acts on both alpha and beta receptors and so can cause peripheral vasodilation (a beta effect) or vasoconstriction (an alpha effect). Also increases both heart rate and contractility (beta effect). Used during cardiopulmonary resuscitation to stimulate heart activity and raise low blood pressure. It is also used to treat anaphylactic shock
Common side effects: tachycardia, palpitations, anxiety, headache, eye irritation, watering of eyes, dizziness, lightheadedness, facial

flushing, headache, dry mouth, nausea, trembling, insomnia, vomiting, fatigue.

Alendronic acid/Alendronate (bisphosphonate)

Inhibits the release of calcium from bone by interfering with the activity of osteoclasts, thereby reducing the rate of bone turnover. Used in the prophylaxis and treatment of postmenopausal osteoporosis and corticosteroid-induced osteoporosis. Often used in conjunction with calcium tablets.

Common side effects: abdominal distension, abdominal pain, constipation, diarrhoea, dyspepsia, flatulence, headache, oesophageal reactions, regurgitation.

Allopurinol (antigout)

A prophylactic for gout, uric acid and calcium oxalate kidney stones and hyperuricaemia associated with cancer chemotherapy.
Common side effects: rash, nausea, vomiting.

Alteplase (fibrinolytic)

Dissolves thrombi by acting directly on the plasminogen entrapped within the clot. Used to treat acute conditions featuring blood clots, particularly ischaemic stroke within the first 4.5 hours of the onset of symptoms. Also given after a myocardial infarct to dissolve thrombi in the coronary arteries and for acute massive pulmonary embolism.

Common side effects: superficial bleeding at puncture sites, hypotension.

Amantadine (antiviral with dopamine activity)

Used to treat mild Parkinson's disease, usually in younger patients, however other treatments are often preferred. Also used for postherpetic neuralgia.

Common side effects: anxiety, dizziness, headaches, nausea, loss of appetite, cognitive impairment, confusion, insomnia, hallucinations.

Amiodarone (antiarrhythmic)

Slows nerve impulses in the heart muscle. Used to treat arrhythmias including paroxysmal supraventricular, nodal and

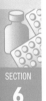

ventricular tachycardias, atrial fibrillation and flutter, ventricular fibrillation, and tachyarrhythmias associated with Wolff-Parkinson-White syndrome.

Common side effects: bradycardia, hyperthyroidism, hypothyroidism, jaundice, nausea, persistent slate grey skin discoloration, phototoxicity, pulmonary toxicity (including pneumonitis and fibrosis), raised serum transaminases, reversible corneal microdeposits (sometimes with night glare), sleep disorders, taste disturbances, tremor, vomiting.

Amitriptyline (tricyclic antidepressant)

Initially developed for depressive illness but no longer recommended. Main use is to treat neuropathic pain and migraine prophylaxis. Also used for abdominal pain or discomfort in patients who have not responded to laxatives, antispasmodics or loperamide.

Common side effects: dizziness, drowsiness, dry mouth, orthostatic hypotension, headache, sweating, weight gain, nausea, fatigue, unpleasant taste, blurred vision.

Amlodipine (calcium channel blocker)

Used to treat hypertension and angina.

Common side effects: abdominal pain, dizziness, fatigue, flushing, leg and ankle swelling, headache, nausea, oedema, palpitations, sleep disturbances.

Amoxicillin (penicillin antibiotic)

Used to treat a variety of infections such as urinary tract infections, otitis media, sinusitis, uncomplicated community-acquired pneumonia, salmonellosis and oral infections.

Common side effects: anaphylaxis, angioedema, diarrhoea, fever, hypersensitivity reactions, joint pain, rash, serum sickness–like reaction, urticaria.

Ampicillin (penicillin antibiotic)

Used to treat a variety of infections such as bronchitis, urinary tract infections, otitis media, sinusitis, uncomplicated community-acquired pneumonia and salmonellosis.

Common side effects: anaphylaxis, angioedema, diarrhoea, fever, hypersensitivity reactions, joint pain, rash, serum sickness–like reaction, urticaria.

Anastrozole (antineoplastic hormone)

Used in the treatment of oestrogen-receptor–positive breast cancer in postmenopausal women.
Common side effects: hot flushes, headache, fatigue, dizziness, joint pain, vaginal dryness, hair thinning, nausea, diarrhoea.

Aspirin (NSAID)

Used as an anti-inflammatory, as an analgesic and to reduce fever. It also inhibits thrombus formation and is used to reduce the risk for heart attack and stroke.
Common side effects: gastric irritation leading to dyspepsia and bleeding, wheezing in aspirin-sensitive asthmatics.

Atenolol (β-adrenoceptor blocker)

Used to treat hypertension, angina and arrhythmias.
Common side effects: hypotension manifested as cold extremities, constipation or diarrhea, sweating, dizziness, fatigue, headache, nausea.

Atorvastatin (statin)

Lowers LDL cholesterol and is prescribed for those who have not responded to diet and lifestyle modification to protect them from cardiovascular disease. Used to prevent cardiovascular events in patients with atherosclerotic cardiovascular disease or diabetes mellitus.
Common side effects: headache, nausea, gastrointestinal disturbances, insomnia, back and joint pain.

Atracurium (neuromuscular blocker)

Used as a muscle relaxant during surgery and intubation and to facilitate intermittent positive pressure breathing in the intensive care unit.
Common side effects: acute myopathy (after prolonged use in intensive care), bronchospasm, hypotension, seizures, skin flushing, tachycardia.

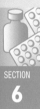

PHARMACOLOGY

Atropine (antimuscarinic)

Relaxes smooth muscle by blocking the action of acetylcholine and is used to treat irritable bowel syndrome. Can be used to paralyze ciliary action and enlarge the pupils during eye examination. Also used to reverse excessive bradycardia, in cardiopulmonary resuscitation and for patients who have been poisoned with organophosphorous anticholinesterase drugs.

Common side effects: constipation, dry mouth, photophobia, reduced bronchial secretions, skin dryness, skin flushing, transient bradycardia (followed by tachycardia, palpitation and arrhythmias), urinary retention, urinary urgency.

Azathioprine (immunosuppressant)

Prevents rejection of transplanted organs by the immune system and in a number of autoimmune and connective tissue diseases (including Crohn's disease, ulcerative colitis, rheumatoid arthritis, polymyositis, systemic lupus erythematosus). Also used to treat severe refractory eczema and myasthenia gravis.

Common side effects: nausea, vomiting, hair loss, loss of appetite.

Azithromycin (macrolide)

A derivative of erythromycin, it is used to treat certain respiratory tract, ear, skin and genital infections.

Common side effects: abdominal discomfort, diarrhoea, nausea, vomiting.

Baclofen (skeletal muscle relaxant)

Acts on the central nervous system to reduce chronic severe spasticity resulting from a number of disorders, including multiple sclerosis, spinal cord injury, brain injury, cerebral palsy or stroke. Common side effects: dizziness, nausea, drowsiness, muscle fatigue/weakness, confusion.

Beclometasone (corticosteroid)

Given by inhaler and used to control asthma in those who do not respond to bronchodilators alone. Also used in creams to treat inflammatory skin disorders and to relieve and prevent symptoms of vasomotor and allergic rhinitis.

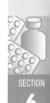

Common side effects: nasal discomfort/irritation, cough, bruising, sore throat/hoarseness, nosebleed.

Bendroflumethiazide (thiazide diuretic)

Used to treat hypertension and oedema.

Common side effects: gout, hypercalcaemia, hyperglycaemia, hyperuricaemia, hypochloraemic alkalosis, hypokalaemia, hypomagnesaemia, hyponatraemia, metabolic and electrolyte disturbances, mild gastrointestinal disturbances, postural hypotension.

Benzylpenicillin (penicillin antibiotic)

Used to treat otitis media, cellulitis, pneumonia, endocarditis, meningitis and throat infections.

Common side effects: anaphylaxis, angioedema, diarrhoea, fever, hypersensitivity reactions, joint pains, rashes, serum sickness–like reaction, urticaria.

Bisoprolol (β-adrenoceptor blocker)

Used to treat hypertension, angina and heart failure.

Common side effects: dizziness, fatigue, cold hands and feet.

Botulinum toxin type A (neurotoxin)

Blocks transmission at the neuromuscular junction by inhibiting acetylcholine release, thereby producing temporary weakness or paralysis of the targeted muscles (approximately 2–3 months). Used to relieve muscle overactivity associated with spasticity and dystonia from various causes, e.g. stroke, multiple sclerosis, cerebral palsy in children, torticollis, chronic migraine, bladder dysfunction. Administered via injection.

Common side effects: pain at site, local weakness.

Budesonide (corticosteroid)

Used as an inhaler in the prophylactic treatment of asthma and COPD. Also given systemically in a controlled-release form for Crohn's disease and ulcerative colitis.

Common side effects: cough, nasal irritation, bruising, sore throat (when used as an inhaler), diarrhea/constipation (when taken orally).

Bumetanide (loop diuretic)

A powerful, fast-acting diuretic used to treat pulmonary oedema due to left ventricular failure. It also reduces oedema and dyspnoea associated with chronic heart failure.

Common side effects: increased urinary frequency and urine volume, muscle cramps, dizziness, hypotension, headache, nausea.

Buprenorphine (opioid with agonist and antagonist properties)

Used to treat moderate to severe pain as well as opioid dependence. Can be administered by injection, sublingually or transdermally (i.e. BuTrans® patch).

Common side effects: sedation, dizziness, nausea, headache, itching at application site, rash, vomiting, constipation, dry mouth.

Calcitonin (salmon) (bone resorption inhibitor)

Regulates bone turnover and is used to treat Paget's disease of bone and hypercalcaemia of malignancy. Also given for prophylaxis of bone loss due to sudden immobility.

Common side effects: abdominal pain, diarrhoea, dizziness, fatigue, flushing, headache, musculoskeletal pain, nausea, taste disturbances, vomiting.

Captopril (ACE inhibitor)

Reduces peripheral vasoconstriction and is used to treat hypertension, congestive heart failure, post–myocardial infarction and diabetic nephropathy.

Common side effects: rash, gastrointestinal disturbance.

Carbamazepine (antiepileptic)

Used to reduce likelihood of generalized tonic-clonic seizures and partial seizure and to relieve neuropathic pain associated with trigeminal neuralgia and diabetic neuropathy. Also used for prophylaxis of bipolar disorder and acute alcohol withdrawal.

Common side effects: dizziness, drowsiness, ataxia, fatigue, blood disorders, rash, urticaria, nausea, vomiting, headache, blurred vision, dry mouth, oedema, fluid retention, increased weight.

Carbimazole (antithyroid drug)

Used to treat hyperthyroidism by reducing the formation of thyroid hormone.

Common side effects: arthralgia, fever, headache, jaundice, malaise, mild gastrointestinal disturbances, nausea, itching, rash, taste disturbances.

Carvedilol (α- and β-blocker)

Used to treat chronic heart failure, hypertension and angina.

Common side effects: fatigue, dizziness, diarrhoea, bradycardia, rhinitis, back pain.

Cefaclor (cephalosporin antibiotic)

Used to treat a variety of infections including acute otitis media, bronchitis, pharyngitis, tonsillitis, respiratory tract and lower urinary tract infections.

Common side effects: oral and vaginal candidiasis, diarrhoea, abdominal cramps.

Cefotaxime (cephalosporin antibiotic)

Used to treat a variety of infections including skin, genitourinary, gynaecological, intraabdominal and lower respiratory tract infections, septicaemia, meningitis and surgical prophylaxis.

Common side effects: oral and vaginal candidiasis, diarrhoea, abdominal cramps.

Cefuroxime (cephalosporin antibiotic)

Used to treat a variety of infections including acute and chronic bronchitis, gonorrhoea, impetigo, early Lyme disease, otitis media, pharyngitis, tonsillitis, sinusitis, surgical prophylaxis and skin and urinary tract infections.

Common side effects: oral and vaginal candidiasis, diarrhoea, abdominal cramps.

Celecoxib (NSAID)

Used to relieve the symptoms of osteoarthritis, rheumatoid arthritis and ankylosing spondylitis. Has a relatively selective action on the inflammatory response compared to other NSAIDs,

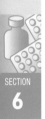

causing less gastrointestinal disturbances. However, it also associated with a greater risk for adverse cardiovascular effects.

Common side effects: dyspnoea, influenza-like symptoms.

Certolizumab pegol (biological DMARD)

Used to treat severe rheumatoid arthritis, psoriatic arthritis, ankylosing spondylitis and non-radiographic axial spondyloarthritis when response to NSAIDs has been inadequate or not tolerated. Given by subcutaneous injection at two-weekly intervals.

Common side effects: hypertension, rash, sensory abnormalities.

Chlorpromazine (antipsychotic)

Has a sedative effect and is used to control the symptoms of schizophrenia and to treat agitation without causing confusion and stupor. Also used to treat nausea and vomiting in terminally ill patients.

Common side effects: drowsiness/lethargy, weight gain, tremor/Parkinsonism, blurred vision, dizziness, fainting.

Ciclosporin (immunosuppressant)

Used to prevent rejection of organ and tissue transplantation. Also used to treat rheumatoid arthritis, and severe resistant psoriasis and dermatitis when other treatments have failed.

Common side effects: gum swelling, excessive hair growth, nausea, vomiting, tremor, headache, muscle cramps.

Cimetidine (anti-ulcer – H₂-receptor antagonist)

Decreases gastric acid production and is used to treat gastric and duodenal ulcers, and for gastrooesophageal reflux disease.
Common side effects: diarrhoea, dizziness, headache.

Ciprofloxacin (antibacterial)

Treats mainly gram-negative infection and some gram-positive infections. Used for chest, intestine and urinary tract infections.
Common side effects: diarrhoea, dizziness, headache, nausea, vomiting, rash/itching.

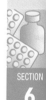

Citalopram (selective serotonin reuptake inhibitor)

Used to treat depressive illness and panic disorder.
Common side effects: constipation, diarrhoea, dyspepsia, nausea, vomiting, indigestion, sexual dysfunction, anxiety, insomnia, headache, tremor, dizziness, drowsiness, dry mouth, sweating.

Clarithromycin (macrolide antibiotic)

Used to treat a variety of infections including bacterial exacerbation of bronchitis, otitis media, acute maxillary sinusitis, pharyngitis, tonsillitis, community-acquired pneumonia, skin and soft-tissue infections. Also used to eradicate *Helicobacter pylori*, responsible for many peptic ulcers.
Common side effects: abdominal discomfort, diarrhoea, nausea, vomiting.

Clomipramine (tricyclic antidepressant)

Used for long-term treatment of depression, especially when associated with phobic and obsessional states.
Common side effects: sexual dysfunction, dry mouth, drowsiness, tremors, dizziness, headache, constipation, fatigue, nausea, sweating, blurred vision, weight gain.

Clonidine (α_2-adrenoceptor agonist)

Used in the prophylaxis of recurrent migraine and to treat hypertension.
Common side effects: dry mouth, drowsiness, dizziness, sedation, constipation.

Clopidogrel (antiplatelet)

Has a similar effect to aspirin on reducing platelet aggregation, although its mechanism of action is different. Prevents arthero-thrombotic events in patients with chronic peripheral arterial disease, recent myocardial infarction or recent ischaemic stroke.
Common side effects: abdominal pain, bleeding disorders (including gastrointestinal and intracranial), diarrhoea, dyspepsia.

Codeine (opioid analgesic)

A mild opioid analgesic that is similar to, but weaker than, morphine. Used to treat mild to moderate pain and is often combined with a nonopioid analgesic such as paracetamol (to form co-codamol). Also used as a cough suppressant and for the short-term control of diarrhoea.

Common side effects: constipation, nausea, vomiting, drowsiness, dizziness.

Co-trimoxazole (antibacterial)

A combination of two antibacterial drugs: trimethoprim and sulfamethoxazole. Used to treat serious urinary tract and respiratory infections which have not responded to other drugs. Also used to treat toxoplasmosis, nocardiasis, typhoid fever and *Pneumocystis* pneumonia and otitis media in children.

Common side effects: headache, nausea, diarrhoea, rash, itching.

Dexamethasone (corticosteroid)

A long-acting corticosteroid that suppresses inflammatory and allergic disorders. Used to diagnose Cushing's disease. Used to treat cerebral oedema, congenital adrenal hyperplasia, nausea and vomiting associated with chemotherapy and various types of shock.

Common side effects: insomnia, facial oedema (moon face), abdominal distention, indigestion, increased appetite, nervousness, facial flushing, sweating.

Diazepam (benzodiazepine)

Has a wide range of uses. Most commonly used to reduce anxiety, relax muscles, promote sleep and in the treatment of alcohol withdrawal. Also used for febrile convulsions and status epilepticus. Dependence develops with prolonged use.

Common side effects: drowsiness, ataxia, dizziness, forgetfulness, confusion.

Didanosine (antiretroviral – NRTI)

Prevents the replication of HIV and therefore the progression of AIDS by blocking the action of the reverse transcriptase enzyme. Usually used in combination with other antiretroviral drugs.

Common side effects: pancreatitis, peripheral neuropathy, headache, insomnia, gastrointestinal upset, fatigue, breathlessness, cough, blood disorders, rash, liver damage.

Diclofenac (NSAID)

Used to relieve mild to moderate pain associated with inflammation such as rheumatoid arthritis, osteoarthritis, ankylosing spondylitis, menstrual pain, moderate headache and musculoskeletal disorders. Also used to treat acute gout and postoperative pain.

Common side effects: headache, abdominal pain, constipation, diarrhoea, nausea, dyspepsia.

Digoxin (cardiac glycoside)

Increases the heart's force of contraction. Used to control breathlessness, tiredness and fluid retention in people with heart failure. Also used to treat supraventricular arrhythmias, particularly atrial fibrillation.

Common side effects: dizziness, headache, diarrhoea, rash, visual disturbances, fatigue, nausea.

Dihydrocodeine (opioid analgesic)

Similar to, but weaker than, morphine and more potent than codeine. Used to relieve moderate to severe acute and chronic pain and is often combined with a nonopioid analgesic such as paracetamol (to form co-dydramol).

Common side effects: constipation, nausea, vomiting, drowsiness, dizziness, headache, dry mouth.

Diltiazem (calcium channel blocker)

Used to prevent and treat angina and to lower high blood pressure.

Common side effects: peripheral oedema (notably of ankles), dizziness, headache, bradycardia, nausea, vomiting, dry mouth, tiredness.

Docusate (stimulant laxative)

Softens faeces by promoting water penetration and retention. Used to treat constipation.

Common side effects: abdominal cramps, diarrhoea (excessive use), hypokalaemia, rash

Dobutamine (inotropic sympathomimetic)

Provides inotropic support in acute severe heart failure, cardiac surgery, cardiomyopathies, septic shock and cardiogenic shock.

Common side effects: tachycardias, hypertension.

Domperidone (antiemetic)

Used to control nausea and vomiting associated with gastroenteritis, chemotherapy or radiotherapy.

Common side effects: drowsiness, dry mouth, malaise.

Donepezil (anticholinesterase)

Inhibits the breakdown of acetylcholine. Used to improve cognitive function in dementia due to Alzheimer's disease, although the underlying disease process is not altered.

Common side effects: gastrointestinal upset, fatigue, insomnia, muscle cramps, urinary incontinence.

Dopamine (inotropic sympathomimetic)

Used to treat cardiogenic shock after myocardial infarction, hypotension after cardiac surgery, acute severe heart failure and to start diuresis in chronic heart failure.

Common side effects: chest pain, dyspnoea, headache, hypotension, nausea, palpitations, tachycardia, vasoconstriction, vomiting.

Dornase alfa (mucolytic)

A synthetic version of a naturally occurring human enzyme that breaks down the DNA content of sputum. Used by inhalation in cystic fibrosis to facilitate expectoration.

Common side effects: rare.

Dosulepin (tricyclic antidepressant)

Used for long-term treatment of depression, especially when associated with agitation, anxiety and insomnia.

Common side effects: drowsiness, dry mouth, sweating, blurred vision.

Doxapram (respiratory stimulant)

Used in hospital to treat acute exacerbations of COPD with type II respiratory failure when ventilation is unavailable or contraindicated.

Possible side effects: arrhythmias, bradycardia, bronchospasm, chest pain, confusion, convulsions, cough, dizziness, dyspnoea, extrasystoles, flushing, hallucinations, headache, hyperactivity, hypertension, incontinence, laryngospasm, muscle spasms, nausea, perineal warmth, pyrexia, tachycardia, urinary retention, vomiting.

Doxazosin (α_1-adrenoceptor antagonist)

Lowers blood pressure by blocking vasoconstrictor sympathetic nerve supply to the small arteries. Used to treat hypertension and to reduce urinary obstruction caused by benign prostatic hyperplasia.

Common side effects: dizziness, tiredness, headache, oedema (particularly ankles), nausea, drowsiness.

Duloxetine (serotonin-noradrenaline reuptake inhibitor)

Used to treat major depressive disorder, generalized anxiety disorder, diabetic neuropathy and stress urinary incontinence.

Common side effects: nausea, dry mouth, constipation, insomnia.

Efavirenz (antiretroviral – nonnucleoside reverse transcriptase inhibitor)

Used to treat HIV infection, specifically HIV type 1 (HIV-1) in combination with other antiretroviral drugs. Not effective for HIV-2.

Common side effects: abdominal pain, abnormal dreams, anxiety, depression, diarrhoea, dizziness, fatigue, headache, impaired concentration, nausea, itching, rash, sleep disturbances, Stevens-Johnson syndrome, vomiting.

Emtricitabine (Nucleoside reverse transcriptase inhibitor)

Used in combination with other antiretroviral drugs to treat HIV infection.

Common side effects: headache, rhinitis, rash, diarrhea, nausea, cough, vomiting, abdominal pain, insomnia, depression, paresthesia, dizziness, peripheral neuropathy, dyspepsia, myalgia, body fat redistribution.

Enalapril (ACE inhibitor)

Used in the treatment of hypertension, chronic heart failure and in the prevention of recurrent myocardial infarction following a heart attack.

Common side effects: headache, dizziness, rash, persistent dry cough.

Enfuvirtide (antiretroviral – entry inhibitor)

Used in combination with other antiretroviral drugs to treat drug-resistant strains of HIV infection. Administered via subcutaneous injection.

Common side effects: acne, anorexia, anxiety, asthenia, conjunctivitis, diabetes mellitus, dry skin, erythema, gastro-oesophageal reflux disease, haematuria, hypertriglyceridaemia, impaired concentration, influenza-like illness, injection-site reactions, irritability, lymphadenopathy, myalgia, nightmares, pancreatitis, peripheral neuropathy, pneumonia, renal calculi, sinusitis, skin papilloma, tremor, vertigo, weight loss.

Epinephrine/adrenaline (sympathomimetic agent)

See Adrenaline.

Erythromycin (macrolide antibiotic)

Used to treat a variety of infections including genitourinary, respiratory tract, skin and oral infections. Also used for Lyme disease and to prevent rheumatic fever. Commonly given to those who are allergic to penicillin.

Common side effects: abdominal discomfort, diarrhoea, nausea, vomiting.

Estradiol (oestrogen for hormone replacement therapy)

A naturally occurring female sex hormone used to treat menopausal and postmenopausal symptoms such as hot flushes, night sweats and vaginal atrophy. Can also be used for the prevention of osteoporosis in high-risk women with early menopause.

Common side effects: withdrawal bleeding, sodium and fluid retention, gastrointestinal upset, weight changes, breast enlargement, venous thromboembolism.

Etanercept (biological DMARD)

Used to treat moderate to severe rheumatoid arthritis, ankylosing spondylitis, juvenile idiopathic arthritis and plaque psoriasis. Given by injection once or twice weekly.

Common side effects: injection site reactions, nausea, abdominal pain, fever, headache.

Etidronate (bisphosphonate)

Inhibits the release of calcium from bone by interfering with the activity of osteoclasts, thereby reducing the rate of bone turnover. Used to treat Paget's disease. Also used together with calcium tablets to treat and prevent postmenopausal osteoporosis and corticosteroid-induced osteoporosis.

Common side effects: gastrointestinal upset, nausea, constipation, increased bone pain in Paget's disease.

Exenatide (antidiabetic)

Acts by mimicking the action of incretin, a natural hormone that boosts insulin secretion and reduces glucagon secretion. Used to treat inadequately controlled type 2 diabetes in combination with other antidiabetic drugs. Administered via subcutaneous injection.

Common side effects: nausea, vomiting, diarrhoea, reduced appetite, weight loss, dizziness, headache, sweating.

Fentanyl (opioid analgesic)

Used to depress respiration in patients needing prolonged assisted ventilation. Also used as an analgesic during surgery and to enhance anaesthesia. Used transdermally to treat chronic intractable pain as well as breakthrough pain in patients receiving opioid therapy for chronic cancer pain.

Common side effects: drowsiness, nausea, vomiting, constipation, dizziness, dry mouth, headache.

Ferrous sulphate (iron salt)

Used to treat iron-deficiency anaemia.

Common side effects: nausea, epigastric pain, constipation or diarrhoea, darkening of faeces.

Flucloxacillin (penicillin antibiotic)

Used to treat staphylococcal infections including pneumonia, ear infections, cellulitis, osteomyelitis, endocarditis, impetigo and for surgical prophylaxis.

Common side effects: anaphylaxis, angioedema, diarrhoea, fever, hypersensitivity reactions, joint pain, rash, serum sickness–like reaction, urticaria.

Fluoxetine (selective serotonin reuptake inhibitor)

More commonly known by its brand name, Prozac, it increases serotonin levels and is used to treat depressive illness, obsessive-compulsive disorder and bulimia nervosa.

Common side effects: headache, nervousness, insomnia, anxiety, nausea, diarrhoea, decreased appetite.

Furosemide/frusemide (loop diuretic)

A powerful, fast-acting diuretic that is used in emergencies to reduce acute pulmonary oedema secondary to left ventricular failure. It reduces oedema associated with chronic heart failure and certain lung, liver and kidney disorders. It is also used to treat resistant hypertension.

Common side effects: increased urinary frequency/volume, nausea, dizziness, muscle cramps, abdominal disturbances, headache, diarrhoea, constipation, electrolyte disturbances.

Gabapentin (anticonvulsant)

Used as an adjunct in the treatment of partial onset seizures, with or without secondary generalization. Can also be used to treat peripheral neuropathic pain and for migraine prophylaxis.

Common side effects: drowsiness, dizziness, ataxia, nystagmus, tremor, diplopia, gastrointestinal upset, peripheral oedema, amnesia, paraesthesia.

Gentamicin (aminoglycoside antibiotic)

Used to treat a variety of serious infections including septicaemia, meningitis, biliary-tract infection, acute pyelonephritis, endocarditis, pneumonia in hospital patients, prostatitis, eye and ear infections, central nervous system infections and surgical prophylaxis.

Common side effects: rare but could include colitis, electrolyte disturbances, hypocalcaemia, hypokalaemia, hypomagnesaemia, nausea, peripheral neuropathy, stomatitis, vomiting, auditory damage, impaired neuromuscular transmission, irreversible ototoxicity, nephrotoxicity, transient myasthenic syndrome, vestibular damage.

Glatiramer (immunomodulator)

Reduces the frequency of relapse in relapsing-remitting multiple sclerosis and is used to delay progression of disability. Also used to treat the initial symptoms in patients at high risk for developing multiple sclerosis. Administered via subcutaneous injection.

Common side effects: anxiety, arthralgia, asthenia, back pain, chest pain, constipation, depression, dyspepsia, dyspnoea, flushing, headache, hypersensitivity reactions, hypertonia, influenza-like symptoms, injection-site reactions, lymphadenopathy, nausea, oedema, palpitations, rash, sweating, fainting, tachycardia, tremor.

Gliclazide (sulphonylurea)

Stimulates the production and secretion of insulin and lowers blood sugar levels. Used to treat type 2 diabetes mellitus.

Common side effects: feeling faint, confusion, weakness, tremor, sweating, constipation, diarrhoea, dizziness.

Glyceryl trinitrate/GTN (organic nitrate)

A potent coronary and peripheral vasodilator that is used for the prophylaxis and treatment of angina. Also used to control hypertension, congestive heart failure, unstable angina and myocardial ischaemia after cardiac surgery.

Common side effects: dizziness, postural hypotension, tachycardia, throbbing headache.

Golimumab (biological DMARD)

Used to treat moderate to severe rheumatoid arthritis, psoriatic arthritis, ulcerative colitis and ankylosing spondylitis. Given by injection at four-weekly intervals.

Common side effects: tiredness, dizziness, dyspepsia, hypertension, injection site reactions, upper respiratory tract infection.

Haloperidol (antipsychotic)

Used to control violent and dangerously impulsive behaviour associated with psychotic disorders such as schizophrenia and mania. Also used to control agitation and restlessness, motor tics, intractable hiccups and Tourette's syndrome.

Common side effects: Parkinsonism, acute dystonia, restlessness, drowsiness, postural hypotension.

Heparin (anticoagulant)

Prevents the formation of, and aids the dispersion of, blood clots. Used to treat deep vein thrombosis, pulmonary embolism, unstable angina, and acute occlusion of peripheral arteries. Also used for thromboprophylaxis in medical and surgical patients as well as during haemodialysis.

Common side effects: haemorrhage, thrombocytopenia.

Hydrocortisone (corticosteroid)

Given as replacement therapy for adrenocortical insufficiency (Addison's disease). Suppresses a variety of inflammatory and allergic disorders (e.g. psoriasis, ulcerative colitis, eczema, acute asthma, inflammatory bowel disease, angioedema).

Common side effects: indigestion, weight gain, acne.

Hydroxychloroquine (conventional DMARD)

Used to treat systemic lupus erythematosus, rheumatoid arthritis and dermatological conditions caused or aggravated by sunlight.

Common side effects: gastrointestinal disturbances, headache, itching, rash, skin reactions.

Hyoscine (muscarinic antagonist)

Used to manage motion sickness, giddiness and nausea caused by disturbances of the inner ear and reduce intestinal spasm in irritable bowel syndrome. Used to treat excessive respiratory secretions in palliative care.

Common side effects: drowsiness, dry mouth, blurred vision.

Ibuprofen (NSAID)

Used to reduce pain, stiffness and inflammation associated with conditions such as rheumatoid arthritis, juvenile idiopathic arthritis, osteoarthritis, sprains and other soft-tissue injuries. Also used to treat postoperative pain, headache, migraine, menstrual and dental pain, and fever and pain in children.

Common side effects: heartburn, indigestion, nausea, vomiting.

Imipramine (tricyclic antidepressant)

Less sedating than some other antidepressants, it is used for long-term treatment of depression and also for nocturnal enuresis (bedwetting) in children.

Common side effects: drowsiness, sweating, dry mouth, blurred vision, dizziness, fainting, palpitations, gastrointestinal upset.

Insulin (peptide hormone)

Lowers blood sugar and is given by injection to control type 1 (insulin-dependent) and sometimes type 2 (maturity-onset) diabetes mellitus.

Common side effects: fat hypertrophy at injection site, local reaction at injection site, transient oedema.

Ipratropium (antimuscarinic)

Bronchodilator that is used to treat reversible airways obstruction, particularly in chronic obstructive pulmonary disease. Also used in acute bronchospasm and to treat severe or life-threatening asthma.

Common side effects: constipation, cough, diarrhoea, dry mouth, gastrointestinal motility disorder, headache, sinusitis.

Isosorbide mononitrate (organic nitrate)

A coronary and peripheral vasodilator. Used as a prophylaxis and treatment for angina and as an adjunct in congestive heart failure.

Common side effects: dizziness, postural hypotension, tachycardia, headache.

Ivabradine (sinus node inhibitor)

Acts on the sinoatrial node to slow the heart and reduce myocardial oxygen consumption. Used to treat angina in patients with normal sinus rhythm and in mild to severe chronic heart failure when β-blockers are contraindicated or not tolerated.
Common side effects: atrial fibrillation, blurred vision, bradycardia, dizziness, first-degree heart block, headache, phosphenes, ventricular extrasystoles, visual disturbances.

Lactulose (osmotic laxative)

Used to relieve constipation and is also used to treat hepatic encephalopathy.
Common side effects: abdominal discomfort, cramps, flatulence, nausea, vomiting.

Lamivudine (nucleoside reverse transcriptase inhibitor)

One of the most common NRTIs for treating HIV infection in combination with other antiretroviral drugs, owing to its excellent tolerance profile. Also used in chronic hepatitis B.
Common side effects: headache, nausea, malaise, fatigue, nasal disturbances, diarrhoea, cough, musculoskeletal pain, neuropathy, insomnia, anorexia, dizziness, fever, chills.

Lansoprazole (proton-pump inhibitor)

Reduces the amount of acid produced by the stomach, and is used to treat stomach and duodenal ulcers as well as gastro-oesophageal reflux and oesophagitis.
Common side effects: abdominal pain, constipation, diarrhoea, flatulence, gastrointestinal disturbances, headache, nausea, vomiting.

Leflunomide (conventional DMARD)

Used to treat moderate to severe rheumatoid arthritis and psoriatic arthritis.
Common side effects: abdominal pain, alopecia, anorexia, tiredness, diarrhoea, dizziness, dry skin, headache, increased blood

pressure, leucopenia, nausea, oral mucosal disorders, paraesthesia, itching, rash, tenosynovitis, vomiting.

Levodopa/L-dopa (dopamine precursor)

Used to treat idiopathic Parkinson's disease by replacing the depleted dopamine in the brain. It is combined with an inhibitor such as carbidopa (to form co-careldopa) or benserazide (to form co-beneldopa) to prolong and enhance its action. It becomes less effective with continued use.

Common side effects: nausea, vomiting, abdominal pain, anorexia, postural hypotension, dysrhythmias, dizziness, discoloration of urine and other bodily fluids, abnormal involuntary movements, nervousness, agitation.

Levothyroxine (thyroid hormone)

Used in the treatment of hypothyroidism.

Common side effects: rare but at excessive dosage can cause cardiac arrhythmias, tachycardia, anxiety, weight loss, muscular weakness and cramps, sweating, diarrhoea.

Lidocaine/lignocaine (local anaesthetic, class I antiarrhythmic agent)

Used as a local anaesthetic both topically and subcutaneously. Also used for ventricular dysrhythmias, especially following myocardial infarction.

Common side effects: injection site irritation.

Lisinopril (ACE inhibitor)

Vasodilator that is used to treat hypertension, congestive heart failure and following myocardial infarction. Also used to treat renal complications of diabetes mellitus.

Common side effects: rash, dry cough, headache, dizziness, postural hypotension.

Lithium (antimanic)

Used to prevent and treat mania, bipolar disorders, recurrent depression and aggressive or self-harming behaviour.

Common side effects: increase in urine, thirst, nausea, fine tremor.

Loperamide (antimotility)

Inhibits peristalsis and prevents the loss of water and electrolytes. Used to treat acute and chronic diarrhoea and faecal incontinence.
Common side effects: dizziness, flatulence, headache, nausea.

Losartan (angiotensin-II receptor antagonist)

Shares similar properties to ACE inhibitors and is used to treat hypertension, heart failure and diabetic neuropathy. Does not cause a persistent dry cough, which commonly complicates ACE inhibitor therapy.
Common side effects: dizziness, diarrhoea, headache.

Macrogols (osmotic laxative)

Softens faeces by increasing the amount of water in the large bowel. Used to treat chronic constipation and faecal impaction.
Common side effects: abdominal distension and pain, nausea, flatulence.

Mannitol (osmotic diuretic)

Reduces cerebral oedema and therefore intracranial pressure. Used preoperatively to reduce intraocular pressure in glaucoma. Also used in the treatment of cystic fibrosis as an adjunct to standard care.
Common side effects: cough, haemoptysis, headache, pharyngolaryngeal pain, throat irritation, vomiting, wheezing.

Maraviroc (antiretroviral – entry inhibitor)

Used in the treatment of HIV infection. Used in combination with other antiretroviral drugs in patients who have a specific drug-resistant strain (CCR5 tropic).
Common side effects: abdominal pain, anaemia, anorexia, depression, diarrhoea, flatulence, headache, insomnia, malaise, nausea, rash.

Meloxicam (NSAID)

Used to relieve the symptoms of rheumatoid arthritis, ankylosing spondylitis, juvenile idiopathic arthritis, and acute episodes of osteoarthritis.

Common side effects: gastrointestinal upset, headache, dizziness, diarrhoea, constipation, rash.

Metformin (biguanide)

Used to treat type 2 diabetes mellitus by decreasing glucose production, increasing peripheral glucose utilization and reducing glucose absorption in the digestive tract.

Common side effects: abdominal pain, anorexia, diarrhoea, nausea, taste disturbances, vomiting.

Methadone (opiate agonist)

Used to treat severe pain. Also used as an adjunct in the treatment of opioid dependence.

Common side effects: drowsiness, nausea, constipation, dizziness.

Methotrexate (cytotoxic and immunosuppressive)

Inhibits DNA, RNA and protein synthesis leading to cell death. Used to treat leukaemia, lymphoma and a number of solid tumours. Also used to treat inflammatory conditions such as rheumatoid arthritis, psoriatic arthritis and Crohn's disease.

Common side effects: nausea, uterine cramps, vomiting, abdominal pain, diarrhoea, dizziness, sweating, tinnitus, bradycardia, chest pain.

Metoclopramide (dopamine antagonist)

Used to treat nausea and vomiting caused by radiotherapy, chemotherapy, opioid treatment, migraines and following surgery.
Common side effects: drowsiness, restlessness, fatigue, lethargy.

Metoprolol (β-blocker)

Used to treat hypertension, angina, arrhythmias and heart failure. Also used in the treatment and prevention of migraine and as an adjunct in the management of hyperthyroidism.

Common side effects: decreased sexual function, drowsiness, insomnia, fatigue.

Metronidazole (antimicrobial)

Used to treat a variety of infections caused by anaerobic bacteria and protozoa including *Clostridium difficile,* pelvic inflammatory disease and eradication of *Helicobacter pylori.*

Common side effects: anorexia, aseptic meningitis, furred tongue, gastrointestinal disturbances, nausea, optic neuropathy, oral mucositis, taste disturbances, vomiting.

Midodrine (α_1-adrenoceptor agonist)

Used for treating severe orthostatic hypotension due to autonomic dysfunction.

Common side effects: chills, dyspepsia, flushing, headache, nausea, paraesthesia, piloerection, itching, rash, stomatitis, supine hypertension, urinary disorders.

Milrinone (phosphodiesterase inhibitor)

A positive inotrope with vasodilating properties, it increases cardiac contractility and reduces vascular resistance. Used to treat severe congestive heart failure and myocardial dysfunction.

Common side effects: ectopic beats, headache, hypotension, supraventricular arrhythmias, ventricular tachycardia.

Morphine (opioid analgesic)

Used to relieve severe pain. Also used to suppress cough in palliative care, myocardial infarction and acute pulmonary oedema.

Common side effects: drowsiness, nausea, vomiting, constipation, dizziness, dry mouth, respiratory depression.

Naloxone (opioid antagonist)

Used for opioid overdose and to reverse respiratory depression caused by opioid analgesics.

Common side effects: dizziness, headache, hypertension, hypotension, nausea, tachycardia, vomiting.

Naproxen (NSAID)

Used to relieve pain and inflammation in rheumatic disease and musculoskeletal disorders. Also used to treat acute gout and menstrual cramps.

Common side effects: gastrointestinal disturbances.

Nevirapine (antiretroviral – non-nucleoside reverse transcriptase inhibitor)

Used to treat HIV infection in combination with other antiretroviral drugs.

Common side effects: abdominal pain, diarrhoea, fatigue, fever, granulocytopenia, headache, hepatitis, hypersensitivity reactions (may involve hepatic reactions and rash), nausea, rash, Stevens-Johnson syndrome, toxic epidermal necrolysis, vomiting.

Nicorandil (potassium-channel activator)

Used for the prevention and treatment of angina. Acts on both the coronary arteries and veins to cause dilation, thus improving blood flow.

Common side effects: headache, flushing, nausea.

Nifedipine (calcium channel blocker)

Used in the treatment and prevention of angina. Also used to treat hypertension, Raynaud's disease and hiccup in palliative care.

Common side effects: tiredness, dizziness, gastrointestinal disturbances, headache, hypotension, lethargy, oedema, palpitations, vasodilatation.

Nimodipine (calcium channel blocker)

Relaxes vascular smooth muscle, acting preferentially on the cerebral arteries. Used to treat ischaemic neurological defects following aneurysmal subarachnoid haemorrhage.

Common side effects: hypotension, peripheral edema, diarrhoea, headache.

Noradrenaline/norepinephrine (sympathomimetic agent)

Administered intravenously to constrict peripheral vessels to raise blood pressure in patients with acute hypotension.

Common side effects: hypertension, headache, bradycardia, arrhythmias, peripheral ischaemia.

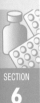

Omeprazole (proton-pump inhibitor)

Reduces the amount of acid produced by the stomach, and is used to treat stomach and duodenal ulcers as well as gastro-oesophageal reflux and oesophagitis.

Common side effects: abdominal pain, constipation, diarrhoea, flatulence, gastrointestinal disturbances, headache, nausea, vomiting.

Ondansetron (serotonin antagonist)

Used to treat nausea and vomiting associated with anticancer drug therapy, radiotherapy and following surgery.

Common side effects: headache, flushing.

Orphenadrine (antimuscarinic)

Blocks the action of the neurotransmitter acetylcholine, and is used to reduce rigidity and tremor (but not tardive dyskinesia) in younger patients with Parkinsonism.

Common side effects: dry mouth/skin, constipation, blurred vision, retention of urine.

Oxybutynin (antimuscarinic)

Reduces unstable contractions of the bladder, thereby increasing its capacity. Used to treat urinary frequency, urgency and incontinence, nocturnal enuresis and neurogenic bladder instability.

Common side effects: dry mouth and eyes, gastrointestinal upset, difficulty in micturition, skin reactions, blurred vision.

Oxycodone (strong opioid analgesic)

Used to treat moderate to severe pain.

Common side effects: drowsiness, dizziness, hypotension, anorexia, diarrhoea, abdominal pain, respiratory depression.

Pancuronium (muscle relaxant)

Long acting, it is used as a muscle relaxant during surgical procedures and to facilitate tracheal intubation. Also used on patients receiving long-term mechanical ventilation.

Common side effects: acute myopathy (after prolonged use in intensive care), hypertension, tachycardia.

Paracetamol (nonopioid analgesic)

Used to treat mild pain and reduce fever. Does not irritate the gastric mucosa, and so can be used by those who have peptic ulcers or can be used in place of aspirin for those who are aspirin-intolerant.

Common side effects: rare but overdose can cause liver failure.

Paroxetine (selective serotonin reuptake inhibitor)

Increases serotonin levels and is used in depression, obsessive-compulsive disorder, panic disorder, social phobia, posttraumatic stress disorder and generalized anxiety disorder.

Common side effects: abdominal pain, constipation, diarrhoea, dyspepsia, gastrointestinal effects, nausea, vomiting.

Phenytoin (anticonvulsant)

Used to treat generalized tonic-clonic seizures, focal seizures and status epilepticus. Also used to prevent seizures associated with severe head injury and neurosurgery.

Common side effects: acne, anorexia, coarsening of facial appearance, constipation, dizziness, drowsiness, overgrowth of gums, headache, increased hair growth, insomnia, nausea, paraesthesia, rash, transient nervousness, tremor, vomiting.

Piroxicam (NSAID)

Has a long duration of action, and is used to relieve the symptoms of rheumatoid arthritis, osteoarthritis, ankylosing spondylitis and for pain relief in musculoskeletal disorders.

Common side effects: gastrointestinal upset, dizziness, headache.

Pizotifen (antimigraine)

Inhibits the action of histamine and serotonin on blood vessels in the brain, and is used in the prevention of vascular headache including classical and common migraines and cluster headache.

Common side effects: dizziness, drowsiness, dry mouth, increased appetite, nausea, weight gain.

Pramipexole (Non-ergot dopamine agonist)

Stimulates dopamine receptors in the striatum and substantia nigra, and is used to treat Parkinson's disease as well as restless legs syndrome.

Common side effects: confusion, constipation, decreased appetite, dizziness, drowsiness, dyskinesia, hallucinations, headache, hyperkinesia, hypotension, nausea, peripheral oedema, postural hypotension, restlessness, sleep disturbances, sudden onset of sleep, visual disturbances, vomiting, weight changes.

Pravastatin (statin)

Lowers LDL cholesterol and is prescribed for those who have not responded to diet and lifestyle modification to protect them from cardiovascular disease.

Common side effects: gastrointestinal upset, headache, fatigue, rarely myositis.

Prednisolone (corticosteroid)

A strong corticosteroid used to suppress inflammatory and allergic disorders, e.g. asthma, chronic obstructive pulmonary disease, eczema, inflammatory bowel disease, rheumatoid arthritis, giant cell arteritis, polymyalgia rheumatica and systemic lupus erythematosus. Also used to treat generalized myasthenia gravis.

Common side effects: indigestion, acne, increased body hair, moon face, hypertension, weight gain/oedema, impaired glucose tolerance, cataract, glaucoma, osteoporosis, peptic ulcer, candida, adrenal suppression.

Pregabalin (anticonvulsant)

Used to treat neuropathic pain, generalized anxiety disorder and also used as an adjunctive therapy for partial epileptic seizures.

Common side effects: dizziness; drowsiness; ataxia; peripheral oedema; weight gain; blurred vision; diplopia, difficulty with concentration, attention, cognition; tremor; dry mouth; headache; constipation; tiredness.

Propranolol (β-blocker)

Used to treat hypertension, angina, arrhythmias, hyperthyroidism, migraine, anxiety and for prophylaxis after myocardial infarction.
Common side effects: fatigue, cold peripheries, bronchoconstriction, bradycardia, heart failure, hypotension, gastrointestinal upset, sleep disturbances.

Quinine (antimalarial)

Used for the treatment of malaria. Also used to prevent nocturnal leg cramps.
Common side effects: tinnitus, headache, blurred vision, confusion, gastrointestinal upset, rash, blood disorders.

Raloxifene (selective oestrogen receptor modulator – SERM)

Used to prevent vertebral fractures in postmenopausal women at increased risk for osteoporosis.
Common side effects: hot flushes, influenza-like symptoms, leg cramps, peripheral oedema.

Raltegravir (antiretroviral – integrase inhibitor)

Used to treat HIV infection in combination with other antiretroviral drugs.
Common side effects: abdominal pain, abnormal dreams, asthenia, depression, diarrhoea, dizziness, dyspepsia, flatulence, headache, hyperactivity, hypertriglyceridaemia, insomnia, nausea, rash, vomiting.

Ramipril (ACE inhibitor)

Used to treat hypertension, heart failure and to preserve kidney function in conditions such as diabetes mellitus. Also used to treat heart failure following myocardial infarction.
Common side effects: nausea, dizziness, headache, dry cough, dry mouth, taste disturbances.

Repaglinide (meglitinide)

Oral, short-acting, antidiabetic drug that lowers blood glucose levels after eating. Used to treat type 2 diabetes mellitus.

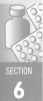

Common side effects: abdominal pain, constipation, diarrhoea, nausea, vomiting.

Rifampicin (antituberculous agent)

Antibacterial used to treat tuberculosis, leprosy and other serious infections such as Legionnaire's disease and osteomyelitis. Used as a prophylactic against meningococcal meningitis and *Haemophilus influenzae* (type b) infection.

Common side effects: red-orange–coloured tears and urine.

Risperidone (antipsychotic)

Used for acute psychiatric disorders and long-term psychotic illness such as schizophrenia, psychosis, mania and persistent aggression in patients with moderate to severe Alzheimer's dementia.

Common side effects: insomnia, agitation, anxiety, headache, weight gain, difficulty in concentrating, tremor.

Ritonavir (antiretroviral – protease inhibitor)

Used in combination with other antiretroviral drugs to treat HIV infection.

Common side effects: gastrointestinal disturbances, headache, rash, liver dysfunction, blood disorders, muscle pain and weakness, metabolic disturbances, cough, anxiety.

Rivastigmine (anticholinesterase)

Used to improve cognitive function in mild to moderate dementia due to Alzheimer's disease and Parkinson's disease.

Common side effects: abdominal pain, agitation, anorexia, anxiety, bradycardia, confusion, diarrhoea, dizziness, drowsiness, dyspepsia, extrapyramidal symptoms, headache, increased salivation, insomnia, malaise, nausea, sweating, tremor, urinary incontinence, vomiting, weight loss, worsening of Parkinson's disease.

Ropinirole (Non-ergot dopamine agonist)

Stimulates the dopamine receptors in the basal ganglia to relieve the symptoms of Parkinson's disease, and has been found to be particularly useful for younger patients. Also used to treat moderate to severe restless legs syndrome.

Common side effects: nausea, dizziness, drowsiness.

Salbutamol (β_2-agonist)

A bronchodilator that is used to treat and prevent asthma, exercise- or allergen-induced bronchospasm and conditions associated with reversible airways obstruction. It is also used in premature labour to relax uterine muscle.

Common side effects: headache, restlessness, nervousness, tremors, nausea, dizziness, throat dryness and irritation, pharyngitis, hypertension, heartburn, transient wheezing.

Salmeterol (β_2-agonist)

A bronchodilator that is used to treat asthma and prevent exercise-induced bronchospasm. It is longer acting than salbutamol and so is useful in preventing nocturnal asthma. It should not be used to relieve acute asthma attacks as it has a slow onset of effect.

Common side effects: headache, cough, tremor, dizziness, vertigo, throat dryness/irritation, pharyngitis.

Saquinavir (antiretroviral – protease inhibitor)

Used to treat HIV infection in combination with other antiretroviral drugs.

Common side effects: gastrointestinal upset, anorexia, hepatic dysfunction, pancreatitis, blood disorders, sleep disturbances, fatigue, headache, dizziness, paraesthesia, myalgia, myositis, taste disturbances, rash, itching, anaphylaxis, peripheral neuropathy and mouth ulcers.

Senna (stimulant laxative)

Used to treat constipation by increasing the response of the colon to normal stimuli.

Common side effects: abdominal cramps, diarrhoea.

Sertraline (selective serotonin reuptake inhibitor)

Used to treat depressive illness, obsessive-compulsive disorder, panic disorder, posttraumatic stress disorder and social anxiety disorder.

Common side effects: abdominal pain, constipation, diarrhoea, dyspepsia, gastrointestinal effects, nausea, vomiting.

Simvastatin (statin)

Lowers LDL cholesterol, and is prescribed for those who have not responded to diet and lifestyle modification to protect them from cardiovascular disease.

Common side effects: gastrointestinal upset, headache, fatigue, rarely myositis.

Sodium valproate (antiepileptic)

Used to treat all types of epilepsy.

Common side effects: temporary hair loss, weight gain, nausea.

Streptokinase (fibrinolytic agent)

An enzyme that dissolves blood clots by acting on the fibrin contained within it. Due to its fast-acting nature, it is useful in treating acute myocardial infarction. Also used to treat other thromboembolic events such as deep-vein thrombosis, pulmonary embolism, acute arterial thromboembolism and central retinal venous or arterial thrombosis.

Common side effects: excessive bleeding, hypotension, nausea, vomiting, allergic reaction.

Sulfasalazine (aminosalicylate)

Used as an antiinflammatory to treat ulcerative colitis and active Crohn's disease. Also found to help in the treatment of rheumatoid arthritis.

Common side effects: abdominal pain, diarrhoea, exacerbation of symptoms of colitis, headache, hypersensitivity reactions, nausea, rash, urticaria, vomiting.

Sumatriptan (selective serotonin agonist)

Used to treat severe acute migraine and cluster headaches.

Common side effects: dizziness, drowsiness, dyspnoea, fatigue, flushing, myalgia, nausea, sensory disturbances, transient increase in blood pressure, vomiting, weakness.

Tamoxifen (anti-oestrogen)

Used in the treatment of oestrogen-receptor–positive breast cancer. Also used in the treatment of infertility due to failure of ovulation.

Common side effects: nausea, vomiting, hot flushes, hair loss, irregular vaginal bleeding and discharge.

Tamsulosin (α-blocker)

Used to treat urinary retention due to benign prostatic hypertrophy.
Common side effects: dizziness, postural hypotension, headache, abnormal ejaculation, drowsiness, palpitations.

Temazepam (benzodiazepine)

Used as a short-term treatment for insomnia and as a premedication before surgery or investigatory procedures.
Common side effects: amnesia, ataxia, confusion, dependence, drowsiness, lightheadedness, muscle weakness, paradoxical increase in aggression.

Tenofovir (antiretroviral – NRTI)

Used in combination with other antiretroviral drugs to treat HIV infection as well as chronic hepatitis B.
Common side effects: gastrointestinal disturbances, headache, insomnia, fatigue, cough, blood disorders, rash, muscle and joint pain.

Terbutaline (β₂-agonist)

Acts as a bronchodilator, and is used to treat and prevent exercise-induced bronchospasm, asthma and other conditions associated with reversible airways obstruction. It is also used to delay premature labour.
Common side effects: nausea, vomiting, fine tremor, restlessness, headache, anxiety.

Teriparatide (parathyroid hormone)

Stimulates osteoblast function, increasing bone density and strength. Used in the treatment of osteoporosis in men and postmenopausal women at increased risk for fractures as well as corticosteroid-induced osteoporosis.
Common side effects: anaemia, arthralgia, tiredness, depression, dizziness, dyspnoea, fatigue, gastrointestinal disorders,

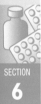

haemorrhoids, headache, increased sweating, muscle cramps, myalgia, nausea, palpitations, reflux, sciatica, vertigo.

Tetracycline (tetracycline antibiotic)

Used to treat a variety of infections including acne, rosacea, diabetic diarrhoea, nongonococcal urethritis, chlamydia and rickettsia.
Common side effects: nausea, vomiting, diarrhoea.

Theophylline (methylxanthine)

Acts as a bronchodilator, and is used to treat acute and chronic asthma and reversible airways obstruction.
Common side effects: gastrointestinal disturbances, insomnia, headache, nausea, vomiting, agitation.

Thiopental (barbiturate)

Used to induce general anaesthesia, as well as reducing intra-cranial pressure in patients whose ventilation is controlled.
Common side effects: arrhythmias, cough, headache, hypersensitivity reaction, hypotension, laryngeal spasm, myocardial depression, rash, sneezing.

Tibolone (hormone replacement therapy)

A synthetic steroid used as a short-term treatment for symptoms of menopause, especially hot flushes. Has both oestrogenic and progestogenic activity. Also used as a second-line preventative treatment for postmenopausal osteoporosis.
Common side effects: abdominal pain, facial hair, leucorrhoea, vaginal bleeding, weight changes.

Timolol (β-blocker)

Used to treat hypertension, angina and for prophylaxis following myocardial infarction. Also commonly administered as eye drops for glaucoma and occasionally given for the prevention of migraine.
Common side effects: lethargy, fatigue, cold peripheries.

Tizanidine (α₂-adrenoceptor agonist)

Acts centrally to reduce muscle spasticity associated with multiple sclerosis or spinal cord injury or disease.

Common side effects: altered liver enzymes, dizziness, drowsiness, dry mouth, fatigue, gastrointestinal disturbances, hypotension, nausea.

Tolterodine (antimuscarinic)

Reduces unstable contractions of the bladder, thereby increasing its capacity. Used to treat urinary frequency, urgency and incontinence.

Common side effects: dry mouth and eyes, gastrointestinal upset, headache, drowsiness.

Tramadol (opioid analgesic)

Used to treat moderate to severe pain.

Common side effects: nausea, vomiting, dry mouth, tiredness, drowsiness, dependence.

Trastuzumab (antineoplastic)

Used in the treatment of HER2 overexpressing breast cancer and stomach cancer.

Common side effects: diarrhoea, weakness, abdominal pain, joint and muscle pain, fever, shivering.

Trazodone (antidepressant)

Used to treat depression and anxiety, particularly when sedation is required.

Common side effects: drowsiness, dry mouth, lightheadedness, dizziness, headache, blurred vision, nausea, vomiting.

Trihexyphenidyl (antimuscarinic)

Blocks the action of the neurotransmitter acetylcholine, and is used to reduce rigidity and tremor. Not useful for bradykinesia.

Common side effects: dry mouth/skin, constipation, blurred vision, retention of urine.

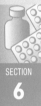

Valsartan (angiotensin-II receptor antagonist)

Shares similar properties to ACE inhibitors, and is used to treat hypertension, heart failure and myocardial infarction with left ventricular failure or systolic dysfunction.
Common side effects: dizziness, renal impairment.

Vancomycin (glycopeptide antibiotic)

Administered intravenously for the treatment of serious infections caused by gram-positive bacteria such as endocarditis, osteomyelitis, septicaemia and soft-tissue infections. Used to prevent infection during surgery when there is a high risk for MRSA. Given orally for the treatment of gastrointestinal infections, notably pseudomembranous colitis caused by the *Clostridium difficile* organism.
Common side effects: nephrotoxicity, ototoxicity (damage to the auditory nerve), blood disorders, renal failure.

Venlafaxine (serotonin and noradrenaline reuptake inhibitor)

Used to treat major depression as well as generalized anxiety and social anxiety disorders.
Common side effects: nausea, dizziness, drowsiness, insomnia, restlessness, constipation, weakness, sexual dysfunction, blurred vision.

Verapamil (calcium channel blocker)

Used in the treatment of hypertension, angina, supraventricular arrhythmias, paroxysmal tachyarrhythmias. Also used to prevent cluster headaches.
Common side effects: constipation.

Warfarin (oral anticoagulant)

Prevention and treatment of pulmonary embolism and deep vein thrombosis. Decreases the risk for transient ischaemic attacks as well as thromboembolism in people with atrial fibrillation, rheumatic heart disease and following artificial heart valve surgery.
Common side effects: haemorrhage, bruising.

Zidovudine (nucleoside and nucleotide reverse transcriptase inhibitor)

Used in combination with other antiretroviral drugs to treat HIV infection. Also used to prevent maternal-fetal HIV transmission.

Common side effects: nausea, vomiting, diarrhoea.

Zopiclone (non-benzodiazepine hypnotic)

Used for short-term treatment of insomnia (up to 4 weeks).

Common side effects: taste disturbances.

Prescription abbreviations

Abbreviation	Latin	English
a.c.	ante cibum	before food
b.d.	bis die	twice a day
nocte	nocte	at night
o.d.	omni die	daily
o.m.	omni mane	in the mornings
o.n.	omni nocte	at night
p.c.	post cibum	after food
p.o.	per os	by mouth
p.r.	per rectum	by rectum
p.r.n.	pro re nata	when required
q.d.s.	quater die sumendum	four times a day
stat.	statim	immediately
t.d.s.	ter die sumendum	three times a day

Further Reading

Hitchings, A., Lonsdale, D., Burrage, D., & Baker, E. (2014). *The top 100 drugs: Clinical pharmacology and practical prescribing* (1st ed.). Churchill Livingstone.

Joint Formulary Committee (2017). *British National Formulary* (74th ed.). London: BMJ Group and Pharmaceutical Press.

Kizior, R. J., & Hodgson, K. J. (2018). *Saunders Nursing drug handbook 2018*. St Louis: Elsevier.

O'Shaughnessy, K. M. (2015). *BMA new guide to medicine and drugs* (9th ed.). London: British Medical Association.

Rang, H. P., Ritter, J. M., Flower, R. J., & Henderson, G. (2015). *Rang and Dale's pharmacology* (8th ed.). Edinburgh: Churchill Livingstone.

SECTION

6

PHARMACOLOGY

Appendices

Laboratory values

Biochemistry

Alanine aminotransferase (ALT)	10–40 U/L
Albumin	36–47 g/L
Alkaline phosphatase	40–125 U/L
Amylase	90–300 U/L
Aspartate aminotransferase (AST)	10–35 U/L
Bicarbonate (arterial)	22–28 mmol/L
Bilirubin (total)	2–17 mmol/L
C-reactive protein	<7 mg/L
Caeruloplasmin	150–600 mg/L
Calcium	2.1–2.6 mmol/L
Chloride	95–105 mmol/L
Cholesterol (total)	Desirable level <5.2 mmol/L
Cholesterol (HDL)	
Men	0.5–1.6 mmol/L
Women	0.6–1.9 mmol/L
Copper	13–24 mmol/L
Creatine kinase (total)	
Men	30–200 U/L
Women	30–150 U/L
Creatinine	55–150 mmol/L
Globulins	24–37 g/L
Glucose (venous blood, fasting)	3.6–5.8 mmol/L
Iron	
Men	14–32 µmol/L
Women	10–28 µmol/L
Iron-binding capacity, total (TIBC)	45–70 µmol/L
Lactate (arterial)	0.3–1.4 mmol/L
Lactate dehydrogenase (total)	230–460 U/L
Lead (adults, whole blood)	<1.7 µmol/L

Magnesium	0.7–1.0 mmol/L
Osmolality	275–290 mmol/kg
Phosphate (fasting)	0.8–1.4 mmol/L
Potassium (serum)	3.6–5.0 mmol/L
Protein (total)	60–80 g/L
Sodium	136–145 mmol/L
Transferrin	2–4 g/L
Triglycerides (fasting)	0.6–1.8 mmol/L
Urate	
Men	0.12–0.42 mmol/L
Women	0.12–0.36 mmol/L
Urea	2.5–6.5 mmol/L
Uric acid	
Men	0.1–0.45 mmol/L
Women	0.09–0.36 mmol/L
Vitamin A	0.7–3.5 µmol/L
Vitamin C	23–57 µmol/L
Zinc	11–22 µmol/L

Haematology

Activated partial thromboplastin time (APTT)	30–40 s
Bleeding time (Ivy)	2–8 min
Erythrocyte sedimentation rate (ESR)	
Adult men	1–10 mm/h
Adult women	3–15 mm/h
Fibrinogen	1.5–4.0 g/L
Folate (serum)	4–18 mg/L
Haemoglobin	
Men	130–180 g/L
	(13–18 g/dL)
Women	115–165 g/L
	(11.5–16.5 g/dL)
International normalized ratio (INR)	0.89–1.10
Mean cell haemoglobin (MCH)	27–32 pg
Mean cell haemoglobin concentration (MCHC)	30–35 g/dL
Mean cell volume (MCV)	78–95 fL

Packed cell volume (PCV or haematocrit)	
Men	0.40–0.54 (40–54%)
Women	0.35–0.47 (35–47%)
Platelets (thrombocytes)	$150–400 \times 10^9$/L
Prothrombin time (PT)	12–16 s
Red blood cells (erythrocytes)	
Men	$4.5–6.5 \times 10^{12}$/L
Women	$3.85–5.30 \times 10^{12}$/L
Reticulocytes	$4.5–6.5 \times 10^{12}$/L
White blood cells (leukocytes)	$4.0–11.0 \times 10^9$/L

Values vary from laboratory to laboratory, depending on testing methods used. These reference ranges should be used as a guide only. All reference ranges apply to adults only; they may differ in children.

Conversions and units

Pounds/kg

lb	kg
1	0.45
2	0.91
3	1.36
4	1.81
5	2.27
6	2.72
7	3.18
8	3.63
9	4.08
10	4.54
11	4.99
12	5.44
13	5.90
14	6.35

SECTION

7

APPENDIX 1

361

Stones/kg

Stones	kg
1	6.35
2	12.70
3	19.05
4	25.40
5	31.75
6	38.10
7	44.45
8	50.80
9	57.15
10	63.50
11	69.85
12	76.20
13	82.55
14	88.90
15	95.25
16	101.60
17	107.95
18	114.30

Mass

1 kilogram (kg) = 2.205 pounds (lb)
1 pound (lb) = 454 milligrams (mg) = 16 ounces (oz)
1 oz = 28.35 grams (g)

Length

1 inch (in.) = 2.54 centimetres (cm)
1 metre (m) = 3.281 feet (ft) = 39.37 in
1 foot (ft) = 30.48 cm = 12 in

Volume

1 litre (L) = 1000 millilitres (mL)
1 pint ≈ 568 mL

Pressure

kPa	mmHg
1	7.5
2	15
4	30
6	45
8	60
10	75
12	90
14	105

1 millimetre of mercury (mmHg) = 0.133 kilopascal (kPa)
1 kilopascal (kPa) = 7.5 mmHg

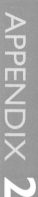

Acronyms and Abbreviations

AAA	abdominal aortic aneurysm
Ab	antibody
ABGs	arterial blood gases
ABI	acquired brain injury/ankle-brachial index
ABPA	allergic bronchopulmonary aspergillosis
ACBT	active cycle of breathing technique
ACE	angiotensin-converting enzyme
ACT	activated clotting time/airway clearance technique/acceptance commitment therapy
ACTH	adrenocorticotrophic hormone
AD	autogenic drainage
ADH	antidiuretic hormone
ADL	activities of daily living
ADR	adverse drug reaction
AE	air entry
AEA	above elbow amputation
AF	atrial fibrillation
AFO	ankle-foot orthosis
Ag	antigen
AGN	acute glomerulonephritis
AHRF	acute hypoxaemic respiratory failure
AI	aortic insufficiency
AIDS	acquired immune deficiency syndrome
AKA	above knee amputation
AL	acute leukaemia
ALD	alcoholic liver disease
ALI	acute lung injury/acute limb ischaemia
ALS	amyotrophic lateral sclerosis
AMI	acute myocardial infarction
AML	acute myeloid leukaemia
AP	anteroposterior
APACHE	acute physiology and chronic health evaluation
ARDS	acute respiratory distress syndrome
ARF	acute renal failure

AROM	active range of movement
AS	ankylosing spondylitis
ASD	atrial septal defect
ATN	acute tubular necrosis
AV	atrioventricular
AVF	arteriovenous fistula
AVR	aortic valve replacement
AVSD	atrioventricular septal defect
BC	breathing control
BE	bacterial endocarditis/barium enema/base excess
BEA	below elbow amputation
BiPAP	bilevel positive airway pressure
BiVAD	biventricular assist device
BKA	below knee amputation
BLS	basic life support
BM	blood glucose monitoring
BMI	body mass index
BO	bowels open
BOS	base of support
BP	blood pressure
BPD	bronchopulmonary dysplasia
BPF	bronchopleural fistula
bpm	beats per minute
BS	bowel sounds/breath sounds
BSA	body surface area
BSO	bilateral salpingo-oophorectomy
BVHF	biventricular heart failure
Ca	carcinoma
CABG	coronary artery bypass graft
CAD	coronary artery disease
CAH	chronic active hepatitis
CAL	chronic airflow limitation
CAO	chronic airways obstruction
CAPD	continuous ambulatory peritoneal dialysis
CAVG	coronary artery vein graft
CAVHF	continuous arterial venous haemofiltration
CBD	common bile duct
CBF	cerebral blood flow
CCF	congestive cardiac failure

CCU	coronary care unit
CDH	congenital dislocation of the hip
CF	cystic fibrosis
CFA	cryptogenic fibrosing alveolitis
CFI	cardiac function index
CHD	coronary heart disease, congenital heart disease
CHF	chronic heart failure
CI	chest infection, confidence interval
CLD	chronic lung disease, chronic liver disease
CML	chronic myeloid leukaemia
CMV	controlled mandatory ventilation/cytomegalovirus
CNS	central nervous system
CO	cardiac output
C/O	complains of
COAD	chronic obstructive airways disease
COLD	chronic obstructive lung disease
COT	continuous oxygen therapy
COPD	chronic obstructive pulmonary disease
CP	cerebral palsy
CPAP	continuous positive airway pressure
CPK	creatine phosphokinase
CPM	continuous passive movements
CPN	community psychiatric nurse
CPP	cerebral perfusion pressure
CPR	cardiopulmonary resuscitation
CRF	chronic renal failure
CRPS	complex regional pain syndrome
CRP	C-reactive protein
CSF	cerebrospinal fluid
CT	computed tomography
CTEV	congenital talipes equinovarus
CV	closing volume
CVA	cerebrovascular accident
CVD	cardiovascular disease
CVP	central venous pressure
CVS	cardiovascular system
CVVHF	continuous veno-venous haemofiltration
CXR	chest X-ray

D&C	dilation and curettage
D/C	discharge
D/W	discussed with
DBE	deep breathing exercises
DDH	developmental dysplasia of the hips
DEXA	dual-energy X-ray absorptiometry
DH	drug history
DHS	dynamic hip screw
DIB	difficulty in breathing
DIC	disseminated intravascular coagulopathy
DIOS	distal intestinal obstruction syndrome
DLCO	diffusing capacity of the lungs for carbon monoxide
DM	diabetes mellitus
DM1	myotonic dystrophy type 1
DMD	Duchenne muscular dystrophy
DN	district nurse
DNA	deoxyribonucleic acid/did not attend
DSA	digital subtraction angiography
DU	duodenal ulcer
DVT	deep vein thrombosis
DXT	deep X-ray therapy
EBV	Epstein-Barr virus
ECG	electrocardiogram/electrocardiography
ECMO	extracorporeal membrane oxygenation
EEG	electroencephalogram
EIA	exercise-induced asthma
EMG	electromyography
ENT	ear, nose and throat
EOR	end of range
Ep	epilepsy
EPAP	expiratory positive airway pressure
EPP	equal pressure points
EP	evoked potentials
ERCP	endoscopic retrograde cholangiopancreatography
ERV	expiratory reserve volume
ESR	erythrocyte sedimentation rate
ESRF	end-stage renal failure
ETCO$_2$	end-tidal carbon dioxide

ET	endotracheal
ETT	endotracheal tube/exercise tolerance test
EUA	examination under anaesthetic
FB	foreign body
FBC	full blood count/fluid balance chart
FDP	fibrin degradation product
FES	functional electrical stimulation
FET	forced expiration technique
FEV_1	forced expiratory volume in 1 second
FFD	fixed flexion deformity
FG	French gauge
FGF	fibroblast growth factor
FH	family history
FHF	fulminant hepatic failure
FiO_2	fraction of inspired oxygen, inspired oxygen concentration
FITT	frequency, intensity, time and type
fMRI	functional magnetic resonance imaging
FRC	functional residual capacity
FROM	full range of movement
FSH	fascioscapulohumeral muscular dystrophy
FVC	forced vital capacity
FWB	full weight-bearing
GA	general anaesthetic/gestational age
GAP	gravity-assisted positioning
GBS	Guillain-Barré syndrome
GCS	Glasgow Coma Scale
GH	general health
GIT	gastrointestinal tract
GOR	gastro-oesophageal reflux
GPB	glossopharyngeal breathing
GTN	glyceryl trinitrate
GU	gastric ulcer/genitourinary
H^+	hydrogen ion
$[H^+]$	hydrogen ion concentration
HAART	highly active antiretroviral therapy
HASO	hip abduction spinal orthosis
Hb	haemoglobin
HC	head circumference

HCP	health-care professional
Hct	haematocrit
HD	haemodialysis, Huntington's disease
HDU	high-dependency unit
HEP	home exercise programme
HF	heart failure/haemofiltration
HFCWO	high-frequency chest wall oscillation
HFJV	high-frequency jet ventilation
HFO	high-frequency oscillation
HFOV	high-frequency oscillatory ventilation
HFPPV	high-frequency positive pressure ventilation
HH	hiatus hernia/home help
HI	head injury
HIV	human immunodeficiency virus
HLA	human leukocyte antigen
HLT	heart-lung transplantation
HME	heat and moisture exchanger
HPC	history of presenting condition
HPOA	hypertrophic pulmonary osteoarthropathy
HR	heart rate
HRR	heart rate reserve
HT	hypertension
I:E ratio	ratio of inspiratory to expiratory time
IABP	intra-aortic balloon pump
ICC	intercostal catheter
ICD	intercostal drain
ICP	intracranial pressure
ICU	intensive care unit
IDC	indwelling catheter
IDDM	insulin-dependent diabetes mellitus
Ig	immunoglobulin
IHD	ischaemic heart disease
ILD	interstitial lung disease
IM	intramedullary
IM/i.m.	intramuscular
IMA	internal mammary artery
IMV	intermittent mandatory ventilation
INR	international normalized ratio
IPAP	inspiratory positive airway pressure

IPPB	intermittent positive pressure breathing
IPPV	intermittent positive pressure ventilation
IPS	inspiratory pressure support
IRV	inspiratory reserve volume
IS	incentive spirometry
ISQ	no change
ITU	intensive therapy unit
IV/i.v.	intravenous
IVB	intervertebral block
IVC	inferior vena cava
IVH	intraventricular haemorrhage
IVI	intravenous infusion
IVOX	intravenacaval oxygenation
IVUS	intravascular ultrasound
JVP	jugular venous pressure
KAFO	knee-ankle-foot orthosis
KO	knee orthosis
LA	local anaesthetic
LAP	left atrial pressure
LBBB	left bundle branch block
LBP	low back pain
LED	light-emitting diode
LFT	liver function test/lung function test
LL	lower limb/lower lobe
LMN	lower motor neurone
LOC	level of consciousness
LOS	length of stay
LP	lumbar puncture
LRTD	lower respiratory tract disease
LSCS	lower segment caesarean section
LTOT	long-term oxygen therapy
LVAD	left ventricular assist device
LVEF	left ventricular ejection fraction
LVF	left ventricular failure
LVRS	lung volume reduction surgery
MAP	mean airway pressure/mean arterial pressure
MAS	minimal access surgery
MCH	mean corpuscular haemoglobin
MC&S	microbiology, culture and sensitivity

MCV	mean corpuscular volume
MD	muscular dystrophy
MDI	metered dose inhaler
MDT	multidisciplinary team
ME	metabolic equivalents/myalgic encephalomyelitis
MEP	maximal expiratory pressure
MHI	manual hyperinflation
MI	myocardial infarction
MIP	maximal inspiratory pressure
ML	middle lobe
MM	muscle
MMAD	mass median aerodynamic diameter
MND	motor neurone disease
MOW	Meals On Wheels
MRI	magnetic resonance imaging
MRSA	methicillin-resistant *Staphylococcus aureus*
MS	mitral stenosis/multiple sclerosis
MSU	midstream urine
MUA	manipulation under anaesthetic
MVO_2	myocardial oxygen consumption
MVR	mitral valve replacement
MVV	maximum voluntary ventilation
NAD	nothing abnormal detected
NAI	nonaccidental injury
NBI	no bony injury
NBL	nondirected bronchial lavage
NBM	nil by mouth
NCPAP	nasal continuous positive airway pressure
NEPV	negative extrathoracic pressure ventilation
NFR	not for resuscitation
NG	nasogastric
NH	nursing home
NICU	neonatal intensive care unit
NIDDM	non–insulin-dependent diabetes mellitus
NIPPV	noninvasive intermittent positive pressure ventilation
NICU	neonatal intensive care unit
NIV	noninvasive ventilation
NNU	neonatal unit

NO	nitric oxide
NOF	neck of femur
NOH	neck of humerus
NOS	not otherwise specified
NP	nasopharyngeal
NPA	nasopharyngeal airway
NPPV	noninvasive positive pressure ventilation
NPV	negative pressure ventilation
NR	nodal rhythm
NREM	non–rapid eye movement
N/S	nursing staff
NSAID	nonsteroidal antiinflammatory drug
NSR	normal sinus rhythm
NWB	non–weight-bearing
OA	oral airway/osteoarthritis
OB	obliterative bronchiolitis
OCD	obsessive-compulsive disorder
OD	overdose
O/E	on examination
OGD	oesophagogastroduodenoscopy
OHFO	oral high-frequency oscillation
OI	oxygen index
OLT	orthotopic liver transplantation
OPD	outpatient department
ORIF	open reduction and internal fixation
OSA	obstructive sleep apnoea
OT	occupational therapist
PA	pernicious anaemia/posteroanterior/pulmonary artery
P_ACO_2	partial pressure of carbon dioxide in alveolar gas
$PaCO_2$	partial pressure of carbon dioxide in arterial blood
PADL	personal activities of daily living
P_AO_2	partial pressure of oxygen in alveolar gas
PaO_2	partial pressure of oxygen in arterial blood
PAP	pulmonary artery pressure
PAWP	pulmonary artery wedge pressure
PBC	primary biliary cirrhosis
PC	presenting condition/pressure control

PCA	patient-controlled analgesia
PCD	primary ciliary dyskinesia
PCIRV	pressure-controlled inverse ratio ventilation
PCO_2	partial pressure of carbon dioxide
PCP	*Pneumocystis carinii* pneumonia
PCPAP	periodic continuous positive airway pressure
PCV	packed cell volume
PCWP	pulmonary capillary wedge pressure
PD	Parkinson's disease/peritoneal dialysis/postural drainage
PD&P	postural drainage and percussion
PDA	patent ductus arteriosus
PE	pulmonary embolus
PEEP	positive end-expiratory pressure
PEF	peak expiratory flow
PEFR	peak expiratory flow rate
PEG	percutaneous endoscopic gastrostomy
PeMax	peak expiratory mouth pressure
PEP	positive expiratory pressure
PET	positron emission tomography
PFC	persistent fetal circulation
PFO	persistent foramen ovale
PHC	pulmonary hypertension crisis
PICC	peripherally inserted central catheter
PICU	paediatric intensive care unit
PID	pelvic inflammatory disease
PIE	pulmonary interstitial emphysema
PIF	peak inspiratory flow
PIFR	peak inspiratory flow rate
PiMax	peak inspiratory mouth pressure
PIP	positive inspiratory pressure
PMH	previous medical history
PMR	percutaneous myocardial revascularization
PN	percussion note
PND	paroxysmal nocturnal dyspnea
PNS	peripheral nervous system
PO_2	partial pressure of oxygen
POMR	problem-oriented medical record
POP	plaster of Paris

PR	pulmonary regurgitation; pulmonary rehabilitation
PRN	as required
PROM	passive range of movement
PRVC	pressure-regulated volume control
PS	pressure support/pulmonary stenosis
PTB	pulmonary tuberculosis
PTCA	percutaneous transluminal coronary angioplasty
PTFE	polytetrafluoroethylene
PTSD	posttraumatic stress disorder
PTT	partial thromboplastin time
PVC	polyvinyl chloride
PVD	peripheral vascular disease
PVH	periventricular haemorrhage
PVL	periventricular leucomalacia
PVR	pulmonary vascular resistance
PWB	partial weight-bearing
QOL	quality of life
RA	rheumatoid arthritis/room air
RAP	right atrial pressure
RBBB	right bundle branch block
RBC	red blood cell
RDS	respiratory distress syndrome
REM	rapid eye movement
RFT	respiratory function test
RH	residential home
RhF	rheumatic fever
RIP	rest in peace
RMT	respiratory muscle training
R/O	removal of
ROM	range of movement
ROP	retinopathy of prematurity
RPE	rating of perceived exertion
RPP	rate pressure product
RR	respiratory rate
RS	respiratory system
RSV	respiratory syncytial virus
RTA	road traffic accident
RV	residual volume

RVF	right ventricular failure
SA	sinoatrial
SAH	subarachnoid haemorrhage
SALT	speech and language therapist
SaO$_2$	arterial oxygen saturation
SB	sinus bradycardia/spina bifida
SBE	subacute bacterial endocarditis
SCI	spinal cord injury
SDH	subdural haematoma
SG$_{AW}$	specific airway conductance
SH	social history
SIMV	synchronized intermittent mandatory ventilation
SIRS	systemic inflammatory response syndrome
SLAP	superior labrum, anterior and posterior
SLE	systemic lupus erythematosus
SLR	straight leg raise
SMA	spinal muscle atrophy
SN	Swedish nose
SNS	sympathetic nervous system
SOA	swelling of ankles
SOAP notes	subjective, objective, assessment, plan
SOB	shortness of breath
SOBAR	short of breath at rest
SOBOE	short of breath on exertion
SOOB	sit out of bed
SpO$_2$	pulse oximetry arterial oxygen saturation
SpR	special registrar
SPS	single point stick
SR	sinus rhythm
SS	social services
ST	sinus tachycardia
SV	self-ventilating/stroke volume
SVC	superior vena cava
SVD	spontaneous vaginal delivery
SVG	saphenous vein graft
SVO$_2$	mixed venous oxygen saturation
SVR	systemic vascular resistance
SVT	supraventricular tachycardia
SW	social worker

T21	trisomy 21 (Down syndrome)
TAA	thoracic aortic aneurysm
TAH	total abdominal hysterectomy
TAVR	tissue atrial valve repair
TB	tuberculosis
TBI	traumatic brain injury
$TcCO_2$	transcutaneous carbon dioxide
TcO_2	transcutaneous oxygen
TED	thromboembolic deterrent
TEE	thoracic expansion exercises
TENS	transcutaneous electrical nerve stimulation
TFA	transfemoral arteriogram
TGA	transposition of the great arteries
THR	total hip replacement
TIA	transient ischaemic attack
TKA	through knee amputation
TKR	total knee replacement
TLC	total lung capacity
TLCO	transfer factor in lung of carbon monoxide
TLSO	thoracolumbar spinal orthosis
TM	tracheostomy mask
TMR	transmyocardial revascularization
TMVR	tissue mitral valve repair
TOP	termination of pregnancy
TPN	total parenteral nutrition
TPR	temperature, pulse and respiration
TURBT	transurethral resection of bladder tumour
TURP	transurethral resection of prostate
TV	tidal volume
TWB	touch weight-bearing
Tx	transplant
U&E	urea and electrolytes
UAO	upper airway obstruction
UAS	upper abdominal surgery
UL	upper limb/upper lobe
UMN	upper motor neurone
URTI	upper respiratory tract infection
USS	ultrasound scan
UTI	urinary tract infection

V	ventilation
V_a	alveolar ventilation/alveolar volume
VAD	ventricular assist device
VAS	visual analogue scale
VATS	video-assisted thoracoscopy surgery
VBG	venous blood gas
VC	vital capacity/volume control
VCV	volume control/cycled ventilation
V_E	minute ventilation
VE	ventricular ectopics
VEGF	vascular endothelial growth factor
VER	visual evoked response
VF	ventricular fibrillation/vocal fremitus
V/P shunt	ventricular peritoneal shunt
V/Q	ventilation/perfusion ratio
VR	venous return/vocal resonance
VRE	vancomycin-resistant enterococcus
VSD	ventricular septal defect
V_T	tidal volume
VT	ventricular tachycardia
VTE	venous thromboembolism
WBC	white blood count/white blood cell
WCC	white cell count
WOB	work of breathing
W/R	ward round

Prefixes and suffixes

Prefix/suffix	Definition	Example
adeno-	gland	adenoma
-aemia	blood	hyperglycaemia
-algia	pain	neuralgia
angio-	vessel	angiogram
ante-	before	antenatal
arteri-	artery	arteriosclerosis
arthro-	joint	arthroscopy

Prefix/suffix	Definition	Example
-asis	condition	homeostasis
atel-	imperfect	atelectasis
athero-	fatty	atherosclerosis
auto-	self	autoimmunity
baro-	pressure	barotrauma
bi-	two, twice or double	bilateral, biconcave
bili-	bile	bilirubin
-blast	cell	osteoblast
brachi-	arm	brachial artery
brady-	slow	bradycardia
carcin-	cancer	carcinogen
cardio-	heart	cardiology
carpo-	wrist	carpal tunnel
-centesis	to puncture	amniocentesis
cephal-	head	cephalad
cerebro-	brain	cerebrospinal fluid
cervic-	neck	cervical fracture
chol-	bile	cholestasis
chondro-	cartilage	chondromalacia
contra-	against	contraindicated
costo-	rib	costochondral junction
cranio-	skull	craniotomy
cryo-	cold	cryotherapy
cut-	skin	cutaneous
cyano-	blue	cyanosis
cysto-	bladder	cystoscopy
cyto-	cell	cytoplasm
dactyl-	finger	dactylomegaly
derm-	skin	dermatome
diplo-	double	diplopia
dors-	back	dorsum
dys-	difficult	dyspnoea
-ectasis	dilatation	bronchiectasis

Prefix/suffix	Definition	Example
ecto-	outside	ectoplasm
-ectomy	excision	appendectomy
encephalo-	brain	encephalitis
endo-	within	endochondral
entero-	intestine	enterotomy
erythro-	red	erythrocyte
extra-	outside	extrapyramidal
ferro-	iron	ferrous sulphate
gastro-	stomach	gastroenteritis
-genic	producing	iatrogenic
haem-	blood	haematoma
hepato-	liver	hepatectomy
hetero-	dissimilar	heterosexual
homo-	same	homosexual
hydro-	water	hydrotherapy
hyper-	excessive	hyperactive
hypo-	deficiency	hypoxaemia
iatro-	medicine, doctors	iatrogenic
idio-	one's own	idiopathic
infra-	beneath	infrapatellar
inter-	among	interrater
intra-	inside	intrarater
iso-	equal	isotonic
-itis	inflammation	tendinitis
laparo-	loins, abdomen	laparotomy
lipo-	fat	liposuction
-lysis	breakdown	autolysis
macro-	large	macrodactyly
mal-	bad, abnormal	malignant
-malacia	softening	osteomalacia
mammo-	breast	mammogram
mast-	breast	mastectomy
-megalo	enlarged	cardiomegaly

Prefix/suffix	Definition	Example
mening-	membranes	meninges
-morph	form or shape	ectomorph
myel-	spinal cord, marrow	myelitis
myo-	muscle	myotonic
naso-	nose	nasopharyngeal
necro-	death	necrosis
nephr-	kidney	nephritis
oculo-	eyes	monocular
-oid	resembling	marfanoid
oligo-	deficiency	oliguria
-oma	tumour	lymphoma
oophoro-	ovaries	oophorectomy
-opsy	examine	biopsy
-osis	state, condition	nephrosis
osseo-	bone	osseous
osteo-	bone	osteolysis
-ostomy	to form an opening	colostomy
oto-	ear	otalgia
-otomy	to make a cut	osteotomy
para-	beside	paraspinal
-penia	deficiency	thrombocytopenia
peri-	around	periosteum
phago-	eat, destroy	phagocytosis
pharyngo-	throat	pharyngoscope
-philia	love of	hydrophilia
phleb-	vein	phlebitis
-phobia	fear of	hydrophobia
-plasia	formation	hyperplasia
-plasty	moulding	rhinoplasty
-plegia	paralysis	hemiplegia
pneum-	breath, air	pneumothorax
-pnoea	breathing	dyspnoea
poly-	many	polymyositis

Prefix/suffix	Definition	Example
pseud-	false	pseudoplegia
pyelo-	kidney	pyeloplasty
reno-	kidneys	renography
retro-	behind	retrograde
rhino-	nose	rhinitis
-rrhagia	abnormal flow	haemorrhage
salping-	fallopian tube	salpingostomy
sarco-	flesh	sarcoma
sclero-	hardening	scleroderma
-scopy	examination	endoscopy
somat-	body	somatic
spondyl-	vertebrae	spondylosis
-stasis	stagnation	haemostasis
steno-	narrow	stenosis
-stomy	surgical opening	colostomy
supra-	above	suprapubic
syn-	united with	syndesmosis
tachy-	swift	tachycardia
thoraco-	chest	thoracotomy
thrombo-	clot	thrombolytic
-tomy	incision	gastrostomy
trans-	across	transection
-trophy	growth	hypertrophy
uro-	urine	urology
vaso-	vessel	vasospasm
veno-	vein	venography

National Early Warning Score (NEWS2) for the acutely ill or deteriorating patient

A clinical assessment tool used in acute and ambulance settings to improve the detection of acute clinical illness, risk for deterioration and clinical response in adult patients, including those with sepsis (developed for the National Health Service, UK). The NEWS2 should not be used for children (younger than 16 years of age), pregnant women or those with spinal cord injury.

Physiological parameters	3	2	1	0	1	2	3
Resp rate (per min)	≤8		9–11	12–20		21–24	≥25
SpO₂ Scale 1 (%)	≤91	92–93	94–95	≥96			
SpO₂ Scale 2 (%) Use if target range is 88–92%, e.g. in hypercapnic respiratory failure, under the direction of a qualified clinician.	≤83	84–85	86–87	88–92 ≤93 on air	93–94 on O₂	95–96 on O₂	≥97 on O₂
Air or oxygen?		O₂		Air			
Systolic BP (mmHg)	≤90	91–100	101–110	111–219			≥220
Pulse (per min)	≤40		41–50	51–90	91–110	111–130	≥131
Consciousness or new-onset confusion*				Alert			CVPU
Temperature	≤35.0		35.1–36.0	36.1–38.0	38.1–39.0	≥39.1	

The NEWS2 observation chart is normally colour coded, with scores of 3 coloured red, scores of 2 coloured orange, scores of 1 coloured yellow and scores of 0 being neutral.

*AVPU is a basic assessment of consciousness that identifies the following levels of consciousness:

Alert – patient is awake

Voice – patient responds to verbal stimulation

Pain – patient responds to painful stimulus

Unresponsive – patient is completely unresponsive

On the NEWS2, the AVPU term has been amended to ACVPU, where '**C**' represents new-onset confusion.

Clinical response to the NEWS2 trigger thresholds

NEWS score	Frequency of monitoring	Clinical response
0	Minimum 12 hourly	Continue routine NEWS monitoring.
Total 1–4	Minimum 4–6 hourly	Inform registered nurse, who must assess the patient.
		Registered nurse decides whether increased frequency of monitoring and/or escalation of care are required.
3 in a single parameter	Minimum 1 hourly	Registered nurse to inform the medical team caring for the patient, who will review and decide whether escalation of care is necessary.
Total 5 or more Urgent response threshold	Minimum 1 hourly	Registered nurse to immediately inform the medical team caring for the patient.
		Registered nurse to request urgent assessment by a clinician or team with core competencies in the care of acutely ill patients.
		Clinical care in an environment with monitoring facilities.
Total 7 or more Emergency response threshold	Continuous monitoring of vital signs	Registered nurse to immediately inform the medical team caring for the patient. This should be at least at Specialist Registrar level.
		Emergency assessment by a team with critical care competencies, including practitioner(s) with advanced airway management skills.
		Consider transfer of care to a level 2 or 3 clinical care facility, i.e. HDU or ITU.
		Clinical care in an environment with monitoring facilities.

Royal College of Physicians 2017 National Early Warning Score (NEWS) 2: Standardising the assessment of acute-illness severity in the NHS. Updated report of a working party. London, RCP

Adult basic life support sequence

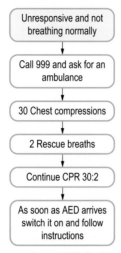

Figure A.1 Resuscitation Council (UK) Guidelines 2015 with permission (www.resus.org.uk)

Paediatric basic life support algorithm (healthcare professionals with a duty to respond)

Unresponsive

↓

Shout for help

↓

Open airway

↓

Not breathing normally

↓

5 Rescue breaths

↓

No signs of life

↓

15 Chest compressions

↓

2 Rescue breaths
15 Chest compressions

↓

Call resuscitation team
(1 min CPR first, if alone)

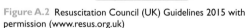

Figure A.2 Resuscitation Council (UK) Guidelines 2015 with permission (www.resus.org.uk)

Index

Page numbers followed by "*f*" indicate figures, and "*t*" indicate tables.

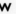